I0025191

"Blending the interpersonal sensitivity of a therapist with the rigor of scientific thinking, Krista Agler speaks to the needs of the human psyche with dexterity, compassion, and sensitivity. Writing clearly, compellingly, and convincingly, she distills the best evidence-based practices from both the therapy room and the science laboratory for dealing with the messiness of life. Read this book and use it to draw from resources you already have so that you can celebrate the victories in your life as well as transform losses into opportunities. Your life will feel easier, freer, lighter, and more joyful when you 'keep in mind' the insights derived from this marvelous book."

Robert Emmons, PhD, editor in chief of *The Journal of Positive Psychology, author of Thanks! How The New Science of Gratitude Can Make You Happier, Gratitude Works* and *The Little Book of Gratitude*

"In this insightful guide, Krista Agler offers a lifeline to those grappling with mental health challenges in today's increasingly stressful world. Drawing from research and clinical experience, she presents a curated collection of evidence-based resources. With its actionable advice and compassionate approach, this is an essential book for anyone navigating their mental health journey. It's a valuable resource that therapists and their clients alike will turn to time and again."

Rotem Brayer, MEd, LPC, author of *The Art and Science of EMDR* and cofounder of The EMDR Learning Community

Keep in Mind

Keep in Mind explores already available resources that makes practical mental health possible for everyone. Taking a holistic approach, the book presents fifteen resources that serve the full spectrum of the human experience. Organized topically for ease of reference, *Keep in Mind* celebrates each resource with research, insight, and inspirational stories.

Bridging the gap between evidence-based data and everyday mental health, *Keep in Mind* offers sixty accessible practices for improving well-being. Readers will come away from the book with increased confidence for pursuing greater mental health, a deeper understanding of the brain-body connection, and a toolbox of readily available resources for building a lifestyle of mental wellness.

Krista Agler is a licensed mental health counselor with a master's degree in professional counseling and over a decade of clinical experience. She is a certified EMDR practitioner and is certified in integrative medicine for mental health.

Keep in Mind

Mental Wellness Resources for Everyone and How to Use Them

Krista Agler

Routledge
Taylor & Francis Group
NEW YORK AND LONDON

Designed cover image: Getty Images

First published 2026
by Routledge
605 Third Avenue, New York, NY 10158

and by Routledge
4 Park Square, Milton Park, Abingdon, Oxon, OX14 4RN

Routledge is an imprint of the Taylor & Francis Group, an informa business

ISBN: 9781032862347 (hbk)
ISBN: 9781032862330 (pbk)
ISBN: 9781003521945 (ebk)

DOI: 10.4324/9781003521945

Typeset in New Baskerville
by Newgen Publishing UK

for Jon,
Eden, Noah, and Simone,
with deep gratitude
and all my love

Contents

Acknowledgments

Keep in Mind has been a passion project of mine for the last few years. It was born in my spare time with the joy of research and discovery and soon grew into an all-encompassing undertaking. It was crafted with the hope of offering something useful. Though it was largely written in solitude, it was not accomplished in isolation. *Keep in Mind* would not be possible without many others and their kind support. In as much as any find solace and practical relief in these pages, I am grateful for the opportunity to put it out in the world and for those who helped it come to be.

And so, I offer my thanks . . .

To the clients I've had over the years, for their willing pursuit of healing, for their trust, and for the honor of partnering together. I count myself privileged to know you, to be a witness to your life, and to walk with you for a little while.

To Rotem Brayer, for his enthusiastic support and optimism, and for offering lights on the runway for publishing. To Dr. Robert Emmons, for mentoring me in gratitude through his work, and for his openness in providing meaningful validation to the work of others, including mine. To Dr. Luke Tse, for advising my first research project in college that ignited passion and joy in study, and for his kind honesty that has improved my work and made it more faithful.

To my Routledge publishing team, for guiding me through the publishing process with patience and clarity. And to Routledge, for championing knowledge and valuing content over trend.

To the experts I have researched and studied, for their commitment to the quality of their work, for their willingness to share information, and for their care for the people who will benefit from their contributions.

I hope my attempt to incorporate too-small portions of your valuable work into accessible practices for all people honors your expertise.

To my beta readers, who first read drafts of *Keep in Mind* and propelled me forward. Your time and energy are imprinted in this book. It may not exist if not for your interest, encouragement, and direction.

To friends and family, for seeing me as a writer and sharing my joy in the process. To those of you who spoke matter-of-factly about the future day I would be published, materializing an experience in my life that may not have been without you. To those who were present in essential moments of deliberation, your keen questions and kind feedback helped keep momentum, inspiring breakthrough. I'm deeply grateful for those exchanges.

To my children, for being living proof of the brilliance that can come through difficulty, for your unabashed celebration of the good wherever you find it, and for the ways you change how others see all people. Eden, Noah, and Simone, you three inspire me to write "for all." I love you three for all of time.

To Jon, my husband, for the practical empowerment that helps others realize their own adventures. Your presence of support throughout writing this book means more than I can say. Thank you for helping create and protect the space for me to do this work. I am most grateful for you. I admire you, and I love you.

To you, the reader, for turning these pages. May you be well, and may you keep in mind . . .

Preface

I have long had the suspicion, and it has grown into a conviction, that being mentally healthy is not beyond our reach and is not a territory for other people or organizations to claim as their own. There is overwhelming force in resources available to each of us to cultivate mental health and realize noticeable relief.

I am a mental health therapist. I don't spend my days in a lab or in academia. I spend my days, hour after hour, with real individual people looking to make real changes in their lives. *Keep in Mind* exists to rally around those needs and honor the desire for change with tangible support. The information provided is not exhaustive, but it is offered as a demonstration of the factual, reliable usefulness of each resource presented.

The priority of practical, accessible mental health began for me at a young age with personal experience. It grew with curiosity over years as a clinical mental health therapist. It became an absolute essential during the mental health ripple effects of the pandemic, with "essential" mental health services available only to some. It has become a determined conviction as I live through my own hardships in tandem with providing ongoing therapy for survivors of the unspeakable. The conviction is this: every person has the right to confidently pursue mental wellness with resources that are available to all.

My first depressive episode came when I was a junior in high school, and it came upon me in a moment. I remember where I was standing when it felt like my brain deserted and joined a team other than mine. The ability to connect with the good around me vanished. The atmosphere seemed to be colder and darker. My stomach sank – and seemed to plummet continually. In the coming weeks, I dissolved. Daily I woke up nauseous, just sick of being alive. I felt numb, yet tears came constantly. Appetite scattered. Friends became distant. I was interested in nothing, and nothing I did seemed to help. I walked around my house as if in a fishbowl, unable to connect with my surroundings. I despaired of life.

Then, one night at dinner, through the fog, I heard my eight-year-old sister ask my mom what was wrong with me. I don't remember the response, but a faint spark went off in my brain. I was reminded that I was not alone in the world and that all that was happening within me didn't just affect me. In that moment I knew, for all I couldn't know for myself, that I did not want my sister's narrative to be that sadness is unconquerable. I resolved then, simply and unemotionally, to change.

Getting medicated or seeing a counselor never occurred to me at that time – I'm not sure why. Perhaps it wasn't the norm in my community or perhaps none of us thought it was that bad. Regardless, I did not receive professional help. Instead, I sought advice from an eccentric but brilliant teacher at school, who also happened to navigate his own depression. He told me I would have to live through it, and also how this was not an obscure thing. There were ways to live through it. Among other things, he told me I had to eat, I had to move, and I had to build routines to live through it. It took months, about three. Daily repeating the same things and waiting. One morning, my brain came back to me. I had lived through it, or perhaps within it.

Not quite a decade later, I began my work as a mental health therapist. I utilized therapies like dialectical behavior therapy (DBT), cognitive behavioral therapy (CBT), motivational interviewing, and eventually integrative medicine for mental health as well as eye movement desensitization and reprocessing (EMDR). I devoted myself to studying trauma and the brain-body connection. In sessions, I would casually drop tidbits like "drink water" or "have you tried eating protein?" They were mentioned almost in passing, and even I didn't think they were the potent contributions I now know them to be. Repeatedly, I would notice how these tidbits came back with surprising and effective results.

Reading more about these almost-too-simple points led me to a world of neuroscience and practical psychology with unignorable proof that what I dropped, as crumbs from the table of counseling, actually seemed to be the more tangible, and at times more effective, offering. I began making "practical lifestyle" an integral part of my practice, continuing to see observable, sustainable and, best of all, client-dependent progress. A thing of beauty.

It was Hippocrates who said, "healing is a matter of time, but it is also sometimes a matter of opportunity" (Ratcliffe, 2016). Often in mental health, we have the capacity to create such opportunities for healing ourselves. My clients are now used to the "opportunities" I extend to them at the end of many sessions as well as the brief rabbit holes of how and why the brain benefits from these "opportunities." I welcome the skepticism I see in these moments, and I relish the return report of how something so simple could be so helpful.

In the summer of 2020, with the pandemic in full swing and the subsequent life alterations increasingly normalized, other mental health professionals and I were deep in conversations about the already approaching and absolutely unavoidable mental health crisis that would result. The isolation, concern turned into fear, and the loss of control in day-to-day functioning seemed a recipe for increased rates of depression, anxiety, and relational discord, as well as spikes in reports of domestic violence and child abuse. And so it was to be.

On a sweltering July day, a psychologist friend and I walked circles at a local park talking about what our different practices were experiencing in this pandemic climate. She told me of the waiting list her practice had to access therapy, reaching into the hundreds. We commiserated about the pain of individuals coming in droves.

"For all those you turn away, and for all those waiting, what can we do for them?" I asked.

Her reply: "Nothing. There's nothing else we can do."

Although I understand the overwhelm and the reality of the limits of our field, I also knew at that moment: "This is unacceptable." Still, I continued to hear the same view from many clinicians.

In the field of mental health, I think we are far from exhausting the creative problem-solving that is possible to make mental wellness accessible to everyone. Beyond that, there is a problematic narrative about humanity in the idea that without formal mental health services people are without options.

Yes, the world is fraught. And yes, many of us come to a point of real struggle with mental health and general well-being. However, we've sailed past the point if we think therapeutic services or products are the make-or-break factor. I found myself wondering, "Why aren't we telling the full story when it is more realistic and reassuring to do so? Why aren't we connecting people with what they have available to them?" It seemed the first line of defense was consistently outsourced: a medication, a podcast, a therapeutic service. All the while, there remains the simple, yet functional phenomenon of being human with what is already within and around us.

At this point, I was convinced that many – if not all of us – could use a reminder of what is available to us as humans to cultivate mental wellness.

Some months later, I was on the phone with a doctor explaining to me that an already intimidating procedure was going to be expanded to include that removal of two masses of uncertain consistency. She explained the procedure to me, and although she was kind and matter-of-fact, I could hardly imagine submitting to the process. For me, it was not a simple surgery for a few reasons. First, when I was four years old, I went through medical trauma that resulted in decades of panic and phobia. Through the lens of this early experience, my brain reacted to the idea of surgery as imminent danger. Second, the surgery was to address a chronic-pain condition of the reproductive system. For two decades I had lived with, at times, debilitating pain. It is hard to explain to those who've not experienced chronic illness the pang of hoping that it could change, wanting it to be different, yet bracing for hope deferred. Third, the condition being treated was also the cause of, at that time, eight years of infertility. The procedure could potentially result in the resolution of infertility or could result in a final closed door on the possibility of ever getting pregnant. These are high stakes. For all these reasons and some others, the choice to move forward with surgery was also a choice to take me past my then-known limits, a challenge to my mental health.

I had already begun brainstorming, researching, and writing a book (this book) on the human capacity for mental wellness and the accessible resources that make it possible. The months leading up to and following surgery became a sort of laboratory for testing resources for their accessibility, practicality, and efficacy. The resulting data convinced me that these resources should be common knowledge and available to all; my experience compelled me to do what I could to offer them to anyone and everyone. And so *Keep in Mind* came into being.

May we keep in mind that there are resources readily available for mental wellness, and that humans have a built-in instinct to use them.

REFERENCE

Ratcliffe, S. (Ed.). (2016). *Oxford essential quotations* (4th ed.). Oxford University Press.

Introduction

To keep something in mind is to both recall that which you've known before and to hold it at the ready for when it will be useful. The human instinct, even when out of practice, knows how to take what is within reach and translate it into improved mental health. It's a lost skill that can be reclaimed. We see it when those in the most dire of circumstances maintain their identity, their resolution, their resilience, and even their joy. What appears to be an anomaly is a call for all to press on and to reconsider what we've accepted as the normal mental state of humans.

The common birthright of available resources means there is hope for all to mend, to regroup, to rediscover how to live life well. Mental health symptoms may not be so much a complaint as a signal to return to form. The default state of the brain-body connection is a lifestyle of sustainable mental wellness found in simple, though perhaps not easy, shifts. Returning to that state comes from remembering these universal resources and putting them to use.

The ensuing transformation is for all. Access, insurance, ability, means, and personality should not determine who may be well. Hardship, loss, and trauma do not exclude anyone. To be human is to have the potential to yet make change and experience relief. The accurate and evolved perspective is also the compassionate one: all humans have the capacity for mental wellness and have access to what it takes.

RESOURCES FOR HUMANITY

Mental wellness resources are available to almost every single person on the planet. In their availability, they stand in contrast from most resources referenced when people discuss mental help or emotional support. There are many other resources not listed in this book and some are more effective than those presented here. Unwaveringly, the focus here is on resources

DOI: 10.4324/9781003521945-1

that are inherently part of or available to all humanity. Some mental health interventions are only necessary at severe points of suffering, while others are a luxury because they are difficult to access. The following resources are distinct, for they are necessary for day-to-day living but also hold therapeutic potency when applied properly. They are effective inasmuch as they are essential, as helpful as they are commonplace.

In the mental health world, these human-empowering resources get lost in the surges of more formal and novel therapeutic approaches. Too often, we've assumed these elements are common knowledge and so do not speak of them, or we assume mentioning them once is enough. Instead, they should be centerpieces of mental health and discussed regularly, clearly, and directly.

A common theme connects each resource: the human system is built to take the resources available, even in small doses, and convert them into improved mental wellness. Though the focus will be on the resources, the broader context is that the basic functioning of human beings has an advantage. Though there is a fragility to our species, it is a misstep to conclude that our state is innately hazardous. People are fitted with the skills needed to withstand, to prevail, and to grow even within harsh conditions.

DEFINING TERMS

Clearly defining terms is a protective measure to accurately frame these resources and the human system in the proper, hopeful context. The following definitions serve the forthcoming discussions with awareness of human capacity and with the aim of practical mental health.

Mental Health

The term "mental health" goes beyond psychological and/or emotional conditions. A condition-based definition of mental health can lead to all-or-nothing perspectives and places weight on pathology rather than capacity. **Mental health is a fluctuating state of the brain-body connection that can adapt to life variables.**

Though it is a state, it's not ideal to draw general conclusions about mental health based on current experience. As it is a fluid state, we have the constant opportunity to influence its direction. A static perspective of mental health may result in discouragement, apathy, or even resignation. The nature of life is varying and unpredictable, making it ill-advised to have a hardline approach. It is not only possible, it is expected to have unpleasant emotional or mental experiences, even while being in good mental health (Galderisi et al., 2015).

Viewing mental health more as a circular feedback loop with many factors and many variations is more adaptive. Circumstances occur, our brain and body have a reaction, we select judgments, we accordingly initiate a chosen response, and then we observe the next circumstances at play. Mental health is the brain-body state of reactions and responses. It changes constantly and is impacted by our influence.

To be mentally healthy is to have a growing confidence and competence to respond to the challenges of life in a way that is beneficial to the whole self and to others. Though mental health has the potential to be shaped by life events and deteriorated by circumstances, it also has the potential to rise to the occasion of life. Point being, mental health is never set in stone; it is alive and responsive. Humans hold a stewardship of their mental health so it can either be passively shaped by situation or purposefully formed with intention.

Though we typically reduce the term "mental"as having to do with the brain in isolation from the rest of the system, it necessarily refers to what manifests out of the connection between the brain and the body. Our "mental" health is going to be determined by the synergy of the brain-body connection. In the following pages, mental health refers to the brain-body state experienced within the ever-evolving process of life and our response to it.

That being said, not all brokenness of the brain or body equates to brokenness of mental health. Certain physical maladies can negatively impact mental health to be sure (Lal et al., 2022), but it would be the wrong conclusion that all physical limits, sickness, or disability mean poor mental health outcomes. I've observed that at times it is quite the contrary. Disability or physical brokenness can often be the habitat for thriving mental health (Hayward, 2013), as if the brain was built with a device to respond to hardship with hidden strength and resilience, resulting in positive mental health effects.

Mental Wellness

Whereas mental health references our current state without over-simplistic descriptors of "good" or "bad," "mental wellness" is decidedly about our positioning in relation to what is good or adaptive. It is more about process than state, but a process headed in the right direction. **Mental wellness is an intended process of the brain and body toward desirable and beneficial ends.**

Mental wellness is about a process of trajectory, characterized by movement toward what is good (McGroarty, 2021). Now, "good" can be debated, but there are universals of what brings ultimate welfare for ourselves and others. We will each have our own preferences that shape some of that wellness, but the posture is facing toward what befits the human system, brain, body, soul. The aim in mental wellness is to align the self with mindsets, practices, and lifestyles sure to benefit the brain-body system and the surrounding context.

Brain vs Mind

The difference between the brain and mind is not one of mutual exclusivity. They necessarily overlap and are often used interchangeably. Together, they are a shared entity best understood and described by their distinctions.

Consider the terms "house" and "home." The house is the nuts and bolts. The layout. The specs. It's literal and shapes a fair bit of what happens in and around it. It functions. It's physical with observable properties. Alternatively, the home is the tone, quality, and experience within the house. It's an abstraction of the house that may be perceived in a variety of ways. Meet me at my house. Welcome to my home. Two different words used to describe two distinct dynamics of the same essential "thing." So it is with brain and mind.

The brain is the organ within the body, with neurons, neurotransmitters, electrical pulses, and so on (Fishbane, 2007). The brain sustains injuries. The brain also heals. The brain is studied by mapping and testing of many different kinds. You can undergo brain surgery. In referring to the brain, we're often talking about the mechanisms at play in mental health.

The mind is more abstract, the experience and expression of mental health. We think of the mind as we discuss personality, perception, opinions, how we're doing. If the brain deals in quantitative data, discussions of the mind can tend to more qualitative conversations, though of course these aren't hard and fast categories. With the mind, there's nuance and self-report involved. The mind includes yours and others perceptions of your mental health: how it feels to you, and how you observe it impacting your day-to-day life.

Just as the terms house and home have a lot of overlap, the terms "brain" and "mind" at times occupy the same territory. Throughout this book, "brain" will refer more to the observable, mechanistic organ, while "mind" will refer to the perceived experience of the brain-body connection.

ABOUT THE BOOK

Above all, this book is meant to be useful. It is meant to serve a purpose, making practical mental health accessible to all who read it. It has been formatted as such, with a specific goal, an intentional layout, and a singular starting point.

The Goal

The goal of mental health, or what it means to be mentally healthy, is not primarily about getting to a certain state, specifically an idealistic one such as constant calm or unflappability. If all mental upset is viewed as pathological, we may get bogged down in unnecessary self-analysis or even avoid aspects of daily living. On the contrary, a full life of passion, connection, and purpose requires some chance, some challenge. Uncertainty will inevitably cause ripples in mental health.

The goal for mental health is a growing confidence in one's skills to respond adaptively to the inner and outer world. Often, the process of healing leads to more experiences, and growth leads to new ventures. With a proper and compassionate view of mental health, the ups and downs become part of the forward movement – rather than reasons for discouragement. If the aim is process, it is easier to recognize the growing confidence and resilience, even if life circumstances get more interesting, complicated, difficult, or even painful.

The Layout

The layout of the chapters to come, the resources they divulge, and the accompanying practices, is purposeful. The book serves as a simple, thorough reference, taking the research of effective resources, distilling them to a powerful dose, and celebrating their usefulness and accessibility. All people have the ability to invest in their mental health. The research attests to the multifunctional use of available resources and the leaning of the human system to put them to use. The following pages outline important perspectives that help foster hopeful expectation and that encourage people to take steps with what's readily available for their mental wellness in order to live more fully.

Going deep into the neuroscience of all these resources is not possible; however, neuroscience education supports mental health and is increasingly utilized in therapeutic settings for its benefits (Tabibnia, 2024). We can consider mental health in more tangible terms and see our action steps as directly effective when we have some concrete structure associated with it. So, throughout the book, I will offer small windows into some mechanisms of neuroscience connected to the resources. The effect of these resources is not just "in your head," as if imaginary. Practical mental health is not an abstract but an endeavor of real substance. Considering, even briefly, different regions of the brain or the neural connections involved can add a utilitarian perspective that is helpful.

There are many resources suited for and available to humans for optimizing mental health. The book champions fifteen of them, organized into sets of five. Each chapter will focus on one resource and will be so named for ease of reference. The chapter will speak to the nature of the resource to give a fresh view of what may seem a common substance or faculty. Then, the chapter will explain some of the science behind why it works effectively. Finally, each chapter will demonstrate how to make the resource part of everyday life through accessible practices, ranging from passive to active engagement: Meditation Practice, Reflection Practice, Conscious Practice, and Lifestyle Practice. The "Meditation Practice" of each chapter refers you to guided meditations that can be freely accessed at kristaagler.com/book/keepinmind. The meditations provide both audio and visual cues.

The first set of resources are the "Internal Resources," which are those available in the basic mental functioning in all humans. They are Existence, Attention, Will, Thought, and Span. The second set of resources are the "External Resources," which are those that reach beyond the mental and into the physical aspects of the human system. They are Body, Breath, Water, Provision, and Rhythm. The third set of resources are the "Communal Resources," which are those that are accessed and shared beyond the limits of an individual person. They are Gratitude, Village, Soul, Contribution, and Meaning.

I encourage going through the chapters in order as some chapters build on use of previous ones; however, the chapters stand alone and can be referenced as such. The resources are commonplace for the sake of availability, yet I urge you not to allow their ordinariness to inoculate you to the impact they can have. A recommended pace to fully digest the content is focusing on one resource a week, however, go at your own pace. Take time, particularly giving energy to the practices.

The Starting Point

In all of this, the starting point is the human agent: you, your child, your client, your employee, your friend. The watershed experience occurs when the resources are activated by the human system. The resources are not a power unto themselves working on you. They are more like singular elements in a chain reaction; human mechanisms are the catalyst. Between nerves and neurons, muscle movement and the senses, hardship and business as usual, the various states of being human react to the resources properly applied. You are the activating agent.

A person cannot be reduced to their current experience of mental health. The temporary state should not be generalized to a person's identity. You are not your struggle. You are not defined by your loss. You are not the trauma you've suffered, nor the damage you've done. Mental health encapsulates more than what is currently symptomatic. Mental wellness takes into consideration the worst of your experience and weaves it in with potential change and approaching relief. No one is out of options.

Any human, living and breathing, has the capacity to improve mental health from the starting point of simply being human. Within monotony or struggle, you and I host within us mechanisms for taking what's available to us and initiating change.

That people would see the light at the end of the tunnel – and would keep moving forward; that our very changefulness would incite courage to try for relief; that incremental healing would be seen as worthwhile; that we could collectively visualize how mental wellness could be a shared experience; that providing for one another from the resources at hand would become the norm; and that no partner, parent, child, marginalized person, victim, survivor, saint, or sinner would think all is lost . . . May we take seriously the resources available and the tool of personhood to pursue practical mental health for all.

REFERENCES

Fishbane, M. D. K. (2007). Wired to connect: Neuroscience, relationships, and therapy. *Family Process, 46*(3), 395–412.

Galderisi, S., Heinz, A., Kastrup, M., Beezhold, J., & Sartorius, N. (2015). Toward a new definition of mental health. *World Psychiatry, 14*(2), 231–233.

Hayward, H. (2013). *Posttraumatic growth and disability: On happiness, positivity, and meaning* [Doctoral dissertation, Harvard University]. Harvard DASH. http://nrs.harvard.edu/urn-3:HUL.InstRepos:11156671

Lal, S., Tremblay, S., Starcevic, D., Mauger-Lavigne, M., & Anaby, D. (2022). Mental health problems among adolescents and young adults with childhood-onset physical disabilities: A scoping review. *Frontiers in Rehabilitation Sciences, 3*, Article 904586.

McGroarty, B. (2021). *Industry research: Defining "mental wellness" vs. "mental health."* Global Wellness Institute.

Tabibnia, G. (2024). Neuroscience education as a tool for improving stress management and resilience. *Current Opinion in Behavioral Sciences, 59*, Article 101401.

PART I

INTERNAL RESOURCES

Chapter 1

Existence: A Resource of Objective Reality and Mindfulness

Simon would say that prior to "the event," he felt normal but not good. Life had not turned out how he expected. Still, he viewed himself as one of the many who had come to the same understanding: this is as good as it gets.

He lost his dad right after he turned eighteen and slowly grew distant from his family afterward, "By my own choice," he recalled. For a few brief years, he pursued intense experiences that made him feel significant. Not inherently risky, but intense. He was part of a band with flash in the pan success that broke apart by the time he was twenty. He got married and divorced before twenty-one. He then got a job with rescue relief crews. It was during one of these assignments that he fell, severely injuring his head. His capacity and sense of self changed overnight. It was life altering; and yet, this was not "the event."

After the fall, he worked as a post worker appreciating the routine. He lived alone, still out of contact with his family, and the days seemed to repeat themselves. Normal, but not good. After ten years, the migraines that began with the fall increased in frequency. He missed work and eventually had to quit altogether.

"The event" came in the middle of the night on the bathroom floor with yet another migraine. He describes the crushing feeling in his skull, the burning behind his eyes, the waves of nausea. Simon readily tells of a moment, when the nausea subsided slightly, and in that moment of relief, he became newly aware of his body, looking at his hands in wonder. It struck him, for the first time, that the fall should have killed him, yet here he was. If nothing else, he was alive and existing in the world. He explains how "the event" of this epiphany altered his perspective, causing him to redefine what it means to be "well," to simplify mercifully, to need help,

DOI: 10.4324/9781003521945-3

and to be present whether in pain or not. In reclaiming his existence, a new way of living became doable.

THE NATURE OF EXISTENCE

To start well, we begin with the most basic, the most foundational. Universally and without exception, existence is a resource for mental health. More than useful, it is essential. The fact of existence as a function of mental health must be stated directly, because it is too often neglected. From my clinical observation, I notice a couple unhelpful trends. First, many of those wanting relief seem convinced that they need someone else to fix them. They are functioning from a belief that they are reliant upon a certain service, medication, therapist, product, or theory. Amid ongoing suffering, there is a posture of waiting for help to arrive. Although feeling helpless is ubiquitous at some point in the human experience, humans are not fundamentally helpless. The second observation is that, after a period of mental illness or inner turmoil, people seem to develop what goes beyond a healthy distrust of the self and moves into territory of viewing oneself as incapable, ruined, or inherently hazardous. In other words, the human system is seen as a liability rather than a primary agent of change that is suitable, versatile, resilient.

To view existence as a resource is to accept some agency, and that can be both overwhelming and relieving. It is overwhelming because it means responsibility – not only some responsibility, but perhaps primary responsibility. The human system is an essential part of the healing process. The help and the resources available require personal activation. The people I have seen truly get well and experience change were those who became active participants in their mental health journey. The brain and body are set up to take part and respond positively. It's not about heroic effort; it's about the logical result that comes with proper use of the system. It's working smarter, not simply harder. Being alive, thinking and moving, having faculties within our control, these are the aspects of existence that make hope for growth, healing, and relief a matter of fact. So, we bear some of the weight of the work needed to change course. The human potential to recover is present even within suffering and not only when all may be well. Helplessness is exhausting and deeply damaging, which is why, I hope, it is also relieving to take in the thought that you can be a primary change agent.

Relief comes, at least in part, in knowing that the wait for help can be over. You are already here, even if it's your suffering that confirms it. Any moment you choose, you can begin or continue movement toward mental wellness. I highlight all the resources named in the pages to come because they are the very resources that are innate to humanity. They are resources you are already using toward some end, perhaps for your mental health and perhaps not. You have existence, and so you have access to resources already available for real, sustainable change. With existence, as with all the resources, starting small is enough to begin.

There is a risk of overlooking the foundational when it is commonplace. Boiling water may be boring, and some may not even consider it a skill, yet it is an essential in cooking. Harnessing existence is the boiling of water in developing a practical lifestyle for mental health. The human system is equipped not only to heal but to be an active participant in that transformation through lifestyle.

It matters how and where we begin. I invite you to begin with your actual existence. Not what you believe about yourself or with how others perceive you. Not with the partial truth that is captured in social media or in one domain of your life. Your actual existence. The word "existence," and its nature as a resource, does not mean the shifting idea of who you are. The word is defined as "the state or fact of having being" (Merriam-Webster, n.d.). Fact. State. Being. Beneath the many philosophies of existence is this foundational fact: you exist.

Objective Reality

Existence is the resource of your objective reality that is foundational to building a practical lifestyle for mental wellness. It is the basic yet changeable context from which we do everything. Objective reality, as relates to our existence, is that which is independent of perception or awareness. It simply is. I am aware that there are broad conversations and generations of literature debating how we define existence and if existence, in fact, exists. In contrast, I'm interested here in a conversation that is painfully practical, to the point of restriction. Acknowledging existence, that state of objective reality, is essential and foundational for mental health.

The objective reality of existence is the basic building block of our being that has to submit to the world we live in, and yet has the ability to uniquely respond. Less preoccupied with tracing the trails left behind or following the trajectory of forward flight, existence is best seen from the point of here and now, as exact as the crosshairs of latitude and longitude. To access the resource of existence, it's necessary to begin at the objective reality of the state of living – now.

Too often we are functioning from a self-concept that is disconnected from present tense, objective reality (Williams and Penman, 2011). Instead, we may perceive ourselves more through our ideas of our reputation, our presentation, or comparison. At times, the comparison can be with ourselves in a different season of life, either positive or negative. Sometimes addressing the past is helpful, certainly. However, there is the essential and too-frequently overlooked component of accurately assessing our current position in order to take effective next steps.

Change as a Function of Existence

By connecting to our existence and beginning with an increased awareness of ourselves as we are, we gain access to potent means for change (Schuman-Olivier et al., 2020). Within our human existence we find other resources that historically and scientifically influence our course of life and how we feel about it. We are not machines with outcomes predicted by input; we are surprising creatures that have a brain- and body-based ability to survive when it seems we shouldn't (Gonzales, 2004). Stories throughout history of underdogs and survivors lay the framework for a narrative available to us all: as long as we still exist the story is not over, and we retain the potential to change.

Some may say that the ones who do well have an exceptional quality that destined them for success. I disagree. After years of clinical observation, I am inclined to see us as more similar than dissimilar and more equal when viewed by our human capacities. There are distinct differences; however, I find them not in essentials but in application. We have similar internal human resources, and we can learn from one another and from history to gently shift the application of those resources for gains in wellness.

Within your existence, you have autonomy. Freedom of existence is certainly different from individual to individual. Where freedom is restricted, the internal resources of a person become even more vital. The impact of external circumstances can be acute; and yet, remaining connected to our objective reality opens up possibilities for response, weathering, and survival.

THE SCIENCE OF EXISTENCE

Using a GPS effectively requires setting the destination. It also requires having an accurate starting point. Most of the time, clients I'm meeting with will have some idea of where they want to end up, even if it's vague. "I want to feel better." "I want to move on." "I want to be happy." However, too often the starting point isn't clearly identified. Instead, it can be a piecemeal idea of who they think they are based on how they see themselves, feel about their lives, compare themselves to others, or how they used to be. We're susceptible to being disconnected from the simple, direct fact of life as it is today. Getting from point A to point B becomes convoluted in the lack of clarity and accuracy of the starting point.

With the expansive, inventive capabilities of the mind, the places I can "be" instead of where I "am" are limitless. There is the ability to consciously shift into daydreaming, the escapism of thinking about something more gratifying than the present. More problematic, perspective can stealthily shift from the present tense self to thinking of ourselves as we were years ago, as others perceive us to be, or as we hope we will be in the future. The concern is not that the picture is necessarily inaccurate, but that forward progress may be limited by the gap between that picture and the reality of the current situation. Indeed, the early phase of therapy often requires a changing of lanes from how a person presents themselves in their day-to-day life to the unadorned truth of how they are *actually* doing. Life change happens in the current moment, in the current self.

Worse still, mental health is disrupted when we associate our existence with our social media account, web presence, or feedback we receive in any nonreal time setting (Carr, 2010). Though you've likely heard it before, it bears repeating, as our minds are too often clouded by missing the stark difference between an actual-now existence and the avatars that go by our names. In the real work of improving mental health, how you present on a screen matters none at all.

The starting point for accessing all other resources for mental health is the actual, here and now, brain-body mechanism in each of us. **Existence provides the neurological basis for a whole-self pursuit of mental wellness.**

Existence, the Brain, and Future Change

Existence is the starting place because the neurological mechanisms involved with human self-concept impact the quality of next steps. The brain is an active player in our experience of existence, or "self-as-object" perspective (D'Argembeau, 2013). It's not just an idea, or a sentimentality of self. The ventromedial prefrontal cortex (vmPFC) is the part of your brain that is functional in planning your next steps, envisioning your future self, and bringing about desired change. It is also a part that is activated in forming your current concept of self. So, activity in this region of the brain is integral to sense of self; sense of self is paramount to forward movement and goal realization (Martone, 2021).

Furthermore, researchers have identified a self-reference effect (SRE), which is the capacity to better remember or recall information due to its relevance to the self (Zhu & Zhang, 2002). As we are conscious of our "self" or existence as we engage in an activity, our brain will associate an increased level of importance to it. Relevant aspects of that activity are more available in the moment and for the future self (Martone, 2021). Furthermore, the objective reality of our existence is understood partially through this SRE and shaped also through first-person subjective experience and perception (Klein, 2012). It is nuanced, to be sure, so the work of bringing clarity is important.

Through conscious self-reference, we strengthen memory and future recall. Future recall is more than what we'll be able to remember in the future; it is also experienced by the brain as remembering something yet to come. How can this be? I don't mean fortune-telling or predicting the future. It's the mental phenomenon of our systems orienting to how we envision ourselves in the future. In other words, we have more clarity of where we want to go and how to get there as we form neural connections in relation to our current self. Returning to the GPS analogy, with an accurate honing of point A (our current self) and point B (where we want to go), the route can correctly connect the two with "future recall," a sort of paving the way. Self-reference is a present tense awareness of our existence that clarifies point A and how we get to point B, priming the routes for change.

In contrast, our brain does not register the past self in mental referencing with the same strength it conceptualizes the self in present and future (Martone, 2021). From a self-reference standpoint, we have more distance at a brain level from our past selves. Still, adverse experiences in the past can affect self-reference in the present, causing a variety of disruptions to mental health (Tian et al., 2021). It's as if the brain is not as activated in present self-reference or proactive future planning when "stuck" holding associations with the adverse past. For this very reason, it is vital and serendipitous that we can actively tap into and strengthen the part of the brain related to self-reference in the present. The question is how. Practically speaking, how do we move forward? How do we reorient from the past self to the current self? For a resource to be practical, we have to be able to actually use it. Enter: interoception.

Interoception

We move now to connect existence in the brain to its expression in the whole person. Though the self-concept connects in the brain, our conscious awareness of it is aided by physical senses. Physical sensations serve extraordinary purpose for mental wellness and accessing all available resources. "A highly symbolic notion like the sense of self is shaped by radically corporeal dimensions" (Monti et al., 2022). Understanding the self through the body happens through a phenomenon called "interoception." It is an essential in mental wellness and will come up again with other resources.

To start, consider interoception's more familiar sister, "exteroception." That word may not ring any bells for you, but it's the term for what we traditionally consider as our senses: sight, hearing, smell, taste, and touch. Through these senses, we can take in what's around us and gain some sense of setting. Interoception comes through the senses of our inner body: heartbeat, respiration, gastric movement, internal muscle contraction, and homeostasis (Monti, et al., 2022). Interoception goes beyond body awareness, which can be pleasant or upsetting, and is characterized by acceptance and a balancing approach (Gibson, 2019).

Interoception, the ability to direct regulating attention to internal senses, can have a "pervasive, stabilizing influence" on the whole self, which includes not only the physical, but also the social, the spiritual, and the mental (Monti et al., 2022). Interoception is central to our awareness and is involved in the activation of that same part of our brain (vmPFC) partially responsible for our sense of self and needed for forward movement. A sense of self involves not only a sense of location through exteroception but also a sense of presence and agency, which are assisted by interoception. The more cued in we are to inner physical sensations through interoception, the more stable our sense of self becomes (D'Argembeau, 2013). The result is more self-discipline, resiliency, coping, among other adaptive faculties (Monti, et al., 2022). Interoception serves multiple purposes such as self-regulation, increasing neural connections, and activating a present tense sense of self. As such, it is helpful in maximizing other resources for mental wellness.

It's possible to have too much of a good thing or an imbalance of a good thing. Too much navel-gazing or self-directed attunement is documented to potentially lead to problematic self-centeredness. Balance is achieved partially through a specific application of interoception. We can engage in interoception with other people through eye contact. Holding another's gaze, even briefly, balances our sense of our own body with the body of another in small, nuanced, hard-to-detect ways that serve as a protective measure against out-of-balance self-awareness (Monti, et al., 2022). The connection isn't through the exteroceptive senses of seeing and hearing and touching; it occurs through imperceptibly tuning the internal senses toward another person.

It follows that an optimal sense of self is part awareness of mental activity (Internal Resources), part embodiment through the physical systems (External Resources), and part connection outside of ourselves (Communal Resources). It just so happens that the resources humans have always had to cultivate mental wellness maximize these very things. Again, beginning with existence is on purpose. The active consideration of the objective reality of the "self" is essential in all that comes next.

Mindfulness: Existence Applied

There is evidence that stepping into a radically present perspective is simply good for the brain (Gibson, 2019). The practice is essential for forward movement as well as the process of healing the brain – quite literally. Most refer to this application of existence as mindfulness, a practice of being purposefully present nonjudgmentally to what is here and now (Williams and Penman, 2011). Now, there is a wide variety of flavors of mindfulness and different routes of practice. Some I have found to be research based and helpful, while others seem to be largely trendy and more appealing than effective. The basics of mindfulness are simple enough in idea, but in practice are countercultural. To practice being, to simply be, to momentarily prioritize objective reality, seems a luxury. I assure you, it is a necessity.

The practice of being present can change "subjective and physiological states" (Smalley and Winston, 2010). In other words, mindfulness alters our physical systems and our mental/emotional experience of life. There are reported positive changes in state, or how people say they feel, that occur while meditating. It goes deeper and longer. Changes have been noted in baseline brain function, reducing anxiety and improving positive mood states with "enduring" change (Davidson, et al., 2003).

Some forms of mindfulness meditation actually increase the amount of grey matter in the brain (Pernet, et al., 2021). Grey matter is in the outermost layer of the brain, or the cortex, which is the wrinkly looking part. It's the part from which we derive our functioning. In fact, it has been found that some of that sought-after cortical thickening occurs in that same part of the brain, the vmPFC, from which we register our sense of self (Yang, et al., 2019). Existence, brain level sense of self, interoception, practicing mindfulness . . . It's all connected and ready to be put to use.

Our ability to function stems from grey matter, which is increased by practicing mindful interoception of the brain-body existence in the actual now. As Plato said, "the beginning is the most important part of the work" (Plato & Bloom, 1968). Starting with existence is paramount in considering any other resource for mental health. When mental health is a struggle, attempting anything to find relief can be overwhelming. By beginning with existence, you can bolster your brain and effectively improve functioning to make all the rest of your resources more available.

EXISTENCE IN PRACTICE

We practice existence through noticing our objective reality in connection with the brain and body in the present. These practices are about beginning well. They are the starting location on the GPS. Practicing the resource of existence is like roots burrowing down to draw nutrients and provide stability for growth. Practicing your actual-now existence will not only be of support to your brain it can also then become a way of living, available in real time.

Existence is present, whether or not we acknowledge its utility to mental health. It can be mistaken as simply our surroundings, the state in which we live, and beyond our influence. In reality, it is both the objective and the subjective self, both open to formation. We get to actively steward it. The following practices serve as opportunities to access the resource of existence and usher in mental wellness as a lifestyle. It may take some time to rediscover that our system has the ability to be authentically animated, here and now.

Meditation Practice – A Guided Meditation on Interoception

As interoception will come into play with many of the resources to come, it is prioritized as our first practice. Following this practice may feel foreign. Or, you may experience it as calming and regulating to your brain-body system. Perhaps both. Regardless, the practice creates and encourages positive connections within the brain and throughout the body. Go to kristaagler.com/book/keepinmind to listen to the provided audio or follow the accompanying prompts for a guided meditation practicing interoception.

Reflection Practice – Self-Reference Reflection to Facilitate Change

As noted, the vmPFC is one pivotal region of the brain associated with our experience of existence and the self-reference effect. The following reflection aims to work with the vmPFC, paving neural pathways for a "future recall" of improved mental wellness. The exercise clarifies and initiates desired change, large or small. Return to the practice as needed with a variety of targets.

Consider: If you were to experience significant improvement to your mental wellness, what would you hope to notice? What would change in your demeanor and day-to-day life? What would it mean to you for that desired change to become fact? Try to frame it in the positive, so instead of "I wouldn't be so angry," consider "I would be more calm." Phrases starting with "I would be . . .," "I will be . . .," or "I can be . . .," may be helpful. Make a brief list of whatever comes up for you.

Whether a single trait or many come to mind, begin with one. If circumstances allow and you're so inclined, say the word or phrase out loud, slowly, three times. In the quiet of your mind, consider what the experience of that trait would be like. Allow yourself to experience the effects of that trait as if it is already accomplished – now. Consider what your posture and facial expression would be if that trait became characteristic of you.

Next, consider a current situation where you would like to demonstrate that trait. Imagine what would be different if you already expressed the desired change. Perhaps thoughts or images of the desired end goal toggle back and forth with your current perception of yourself. Allow these to blend together, noting the starting point of your current, matter-of-fact person. Alternating perspectives between these different versions of yourself allow the "GPS" to prime routes for change, connecting objective reality now with where you want to go.

Conscious Practice – Creating Cues for Mindful Interoception

Developing the skill of interoception begins as a formal practice, but then ideally becomes a part of life. We can aid interoception in this transition by associating the practice with specific cues positioned through our day. It is another application of self-reference. By tuning into the internal senses and doing so at specific times or during specific activities, we create a learned pathway, a neural connection that utilizes existence practically.

We will connect interoception with three-to-five common, daily routines to establish the cues. A couple options: you could select specific times throughout the day and set up alarms or reminders; or, you may pick activities you do each day such as making coffee, brushing teeth, getting in the car, logging in to your work computer, waiting to pick up kids, standing at the bus stop, washing dishes, or turning out the light. Either way, the goal is to pair interoception with the identified time or activity. Very briefly, even ten seconds, acknowledge the present-tense nature of existence in that moment or activity while also engaging in interoception: sensing your heart rate, lungs, stomach, and muscle. Remember, it doesn't have to feel pleasant; it is simply tuning into those internal senses in association with the fact of your objective reality, here and now. Reinforce these cues daily for at least a week. Then, seek out new cues. Aim for cues that span your life, including the mundane, the pleasurable, and the challenging.

Lifestyle Practice – Piloting Daily Existence

As beneficial as regular, formal practice can be, incorporating skills into a way of life holds more longevity. For our purposes, "lifestyle" is a pattern that has become a part of life. Learning to steward existence proactively and even involuntarily helps maintain the mental channels for both immediate balance and long-term changes. Interoception goes with you and becomes a portable resource for regulation from the brain through all parts of your system. The goal is to make interoception a primary, reflexive response to almost any life scenario.

As you go about your life, find ways to tune into internal senses and tangible anchors of objective reality, briefly and frequently. Almost like the spaces between words in a written sentence, momentary check-ins should come often in our responses. Get out of bed, but first, interoception. Write the email, but first, interoception. Get a glass of water, but first, interoception. Say goodbye, but first, interoception. As proper use of existence is foundational in the pursuit of mental health, get in the habit of viewing everything as an indicator to, first, step into the pilot seat of existence. Some daily occurrences that could serve as indicators: boredom or the mind wandering, alarms of any kind, awareness of senses, disruptive physical or mental symptoms, transitions, discomfort or tension, emotions. The routine is not intended to resolve all problems directly; it will, however, ensure that you are starting well in what comes next. First things first.

IN SUMMARY

Your brain and body use a present tense sense of self to posture for beneficial, forward movement. From your prefrontal cortex to the imperceptible feel of your heartbeat in your veins, your objective reality serves to help carry you into wellness. The self-reference effect is one way to practice existence for practical change. Interoception is the ubiquitous skill we can use at any time for truly whole-person benefit. Mindfulness is an effective way to apply existence. Each are brain-building skills that can be utilized on purpose.

The constant presence of our existence while we breathe is the constant opportunity for change. Often, difficulty becomes the catalyst, not the obstacle, for utilizing our existence. Dostoyevsky, after narrowly escaping execution and while still imprisoned, penned the following words in a letter: "Life is a gift . . . Every minute could have been an eternity of happiness! If only youth knew! Now my life will change; now I will be reborn" (1988).

REFERENCES

Carr, N. G. (2010). *The Shallows: What the internet is doing to our brains* (1st ed.). W.W. Norton.

D'Argembeau, A. (2013). On the role of the ventromedial prefrontal cortex in self-processing: the valuation hypothesis. *Frontiers in Human Neuroscience, 7,* 372–372.

Davidson, R. J., Kabat-Zinn, J., Schumacher, J., Rosenkranz, M., Muller, D., Santorelli, S. F., Urbanowski, F., Harrington, A., Bonus, K., & Sheridan, J. F. (2003). Alterations in brain and immune function produced by mindfulness meditation. *Psychosomatic Medicine, 65*(4), 564–570.

Dostoyevsky, F., Lowe, D. A., & Meyer, R. (1988). *Fyodor Dostoevsky: Complete letters: Vol. 1, 1832–1859.* Ardis.

Gibson, J. (2019). Mindfulness, interoception, and the body: A contemporary perspective. *Frontiers in Psychology, 10,* Article 475917.

Gonzales, L. (2004). *Deep survival: who lives, who dies, and why: True stories of miraculous endurance and sudden death* (1st ed.) W. W. Norton & Co.

Greene, R. (2007). *The 33 strategies of war.* Penguin Books.

Klein, S. B. (2012). Self, memory, and the self-reference effect: an examination of conceptual and methodological issues. *Personality and Social Psychology Review, 16*(3), 283–300.

Martone, R. (2021). How our brain preserves our sense of self. *Scientific American.* December 21, 2022.

Merriam-Webster. (n.d.). Existence. In *Merriam-Webster.com dictionary.* Retrieved November 21, 2023.

Monti, A., Porciello, G., Panasiti, M. S., & Aglioti, S. M. (2022). The inside of me: interoceptive constraints on the concept of self in neuroscience and clinical psychology. *Psychological Research, 86*(8), 2468–2477.

Pernet, C. R., Belov, N., Delorme, A., & Zammit, A. (2021). Mindfulness related changes in grey matter: a systematic review and meta-analysis. *Brain Imaging and Behavior, 15*(5), 2720–2730.

Plato, & Bloom, A. (1968). *The Republic.* New York, Basic Books.

Schuman-Olivier, Z., Trombka, M., Lovas, D. A., Brewer, J. A., Vago, D. R., Gawande, R., Dunne, J. P., Lazar, S. W., Loucks, E. B., & Fulwiler, C. (2020). Mindfulness and Behavior Change. *Harvard Review of Psychiatry, 28*(6), 371–394.

Smalley, S. L., & Winston, D. (2010). *Fully present: The science, art, and practice of mindfulness.* Da Capo Press.

Tian, T., Li, J., Zhang, G., Wang, J., Liu, D., Wan, C., Fang, J., Wu, D., Zhou, Y., Zhu, W. (2021). Effects of childhood trauma experience and BDNF Val66Met polymorphism on brain plasticity relate to emotion regulation. *Behavioral Brain Research.* 398, Article 112949.

Williams, M., & Penman, D. (2011). *Mindfulness: An eight-week plan for finding peace in a frantic world.* Rodale Books.

Yang, C.C., Barrós-Loscertales, A., Li, M., Pinazo, D., Borchardt, V., Ávila César, & Walter, M. (2019). Alterations in brain structure and amplitude of low-frequency after 8 weeks of mindfulness meditation training in meditation-naïve subjects. *Scientific Reports, 9*(1), 1–10.

Zhu, Y., & Zhang, L. (2002). An experimental study on the self-reference effect. *Science in China Series C: Life Sciences. 45*, 120–128.

Chapter 2

Attention: A Resource of Selecting Relevance

Nine-year-old Bella was in her seventh foster home. At an early age, she reached the limit of pain and abuse that she could sustain while maintaining functioning. Her behaviors became a constant expression of psychological chaos and traumatic recall. She ran away often. She would try to eat glass and rocks. She couldn't control her bodily functions like most people her age. These behaviors are not uncommon in children like Bella who have experience physical and sexual abuse as well as profound neglect.

When Bella first went to therapy, she was frightened, numbed, and overmedicated. She had a demeanor that, although untrusting, couldn't hide the desire to connect. She wanted to laugh with people, wanted to be noticed for what she did well. Most of the time she seemed half present, blinking often in an internal wrestling of pictures and memories others couldn't see.

Bella felt much safer outside than anywhere indoors, which is why she ran away so often. From her earliest memory, probably shortly after she could walk, she experienced abuse from her caretakers so often she would leave the house and hide outside for hours and sometimes days. In art-projection tests, she communicated clearly that trees were better parents than people. Trees don't hit or violate, and are predictably found right where they were left. She drew people with heavy, jagged, monsterlike lines with flames for eyes and hands, and then trees with long encircling arms, branches sheltering around. She was finally willing to engage in therapy with outdoor sessions. Still, before she could do mindful breathing or grounding practices, she needed a safe foundation. She needed to reclaim her attention.

While walking outside for therapy, Bella learned to isolate each sense and to direct attention to the tangible elements of the present moment.

DOI: 10.4324/9781003521945-4

Directing the senses with attention gave her the capacity to, even momentarily, exit the constant memories. During these walks a shift occurred. Her shoulders dropped and blinking became normal. She would laugh and talk about her favorite things. She was more in the present than in her past. She eventually progressed with trauma treatment. The differentiating factor for her was attention. In casual walks around the parking lot noticing what was in front of her, she developed the ability to direct attention. In learning her attention could be turned from the images in her mind to the security around her, she learned she had an ability to change her experience.

THE NATURE OF ATTENTION

Attention is an ability. It is the essential ability to control the finite processes our brain has to make sense (Lindsay, 2020). It is an ability that differs person-to-person, but it is one that is intrinsic to human beings. Few are the exceptions. To be human is to retain attention. For our purposes, attention is the ability to take notice or to apply the mind. It is how we ascribe mental importance to information, observations, and experiences. People often think of attention through a lens of "attention deficit," or as a problematic part of life when we forget things or become disorganized. Attention as a resource is beyond that.

Defining Attention as an Ability

Attention is a mental resource of ability with which we connect our existence to experience. It is a shift, and an important one, to see attention not as just a function that happens, as if passively, but as an ability. An ability is a skill, and as such it is meant not only to be used, but to be nurtured and maximized for usefulness. It is "characterized by a limited capacity for processing information and that this allocation can be intentionally controlled" (Styles, 2006). It is a skill to take notice, to apply the mind, and to ascribe mental importance.

From birth, humans demonstrate the skill of noticing. All day long, we are noticing. To begin harnessing attention, the task is to take notice, to intentionally control the constant witnessing we do almost in passing.

Humans are also able to apply the mind to varying degrees. Applying the mind refers to devoting our faculties to a task or consideration. It's possible to apply the mind to the work at hand or to scrolling on social media. At times, we apply the mind to proactively listening to our partner, and at other times it is applied to the taste of dinner, a distant memory, or mentally making plans. The mind can be applied to reading the news, to comparison with peers, to replaying past conversations, to attempting a new hobby, to expecting failure, to hoping for the best, and to taking action. Applying the mind involves voluntarily devoting mental real estate to a given direction. And we do it all the time, passively or purposefully.

Attention is also the skill of ascribing mental importance, and this makes all the difference. Behavioral planning is shaped in part by "priority maps" in the brain that are value based (Klink, et al., 2014). Values can be reflective or passive, formed by culture, upbringing, personality, or experience. Values can also be selected, chosen by design toward a specific outcome. Whether driven by default values or deliberate values, our daily living will follow a map. Through attention and selected values, we can ascribe mental importance in a way that changes life. Where mental importance is identified, attention follows. Mental importance can be passively created or proactively selected through values.

THE SCIENCE OF ATTENTION

Attention is the ability to purposefully connect our objective reality with experience, which is the variety of stimulus and information around us. Intentional use of attention builds a bridge between existence and experience. Attention improves mental well-being as it alters the quality and content of the connection between the two. The ability of attention, to varying degrees, is present in each of us (Posner et al., 2020). It is a resource that can be nurtured and strengthened with intentional use. **Attention provides the opportunity to direct focus, creating neural connections that align experience and existence with what matters to us.**

The objective reality of human existence comes into play here as our exteroceptive and interoceptive senses provide key pieces of data used by attention. Attention characterizes the learning and recall involved in shaping our experience of data and informs our response to it (Lindsay, 2020). It is the conscious way we orient to our surroundings, and not just our physical surroundings, but the collective context of input. Body sensations, thoughts, emotions, location, current events, and social interactions are just some of the stimuli making up our surroundings. For the sake of simplicity, I'm going to refer to our conscious awareness of the data coming from our context as "experience."

Inasmuch as our functioning and experience is shaped by our brain, understanding some of the attention processes therein can make the change we're reaching for more tangible. We intervene at an attention level not because it's what you "should" do, like the directive "pay attention" implies. Attention is a resource and an intervention because it works for you and is crucial in moving you the direction you want to go, specifically with mental health.

Attention Networks

Attention works in the brain through three different networks. Think of it like three different forms of transportation in a city. There's ground traffic with cars on the street regulated by stop lights, traffic signs, and so forth. There's the underground subway system, guided by rails. And there's the ferry system, using waterways and channels for conveyance. The three networks are present in the same city space, or your brain, though they occupy slightly different territories. They serve a similar purpose of transportation, or attention, but they do that through different functions. The three functions of attention in your brain are alerting, orienting, and executing (Posner et al., 2020).

The alerting network is responsible for being awake when appropriate, and attentive as needed. It is also responsible for the warning response and the capacity to predict what's coming. It is located in the part of the brainstem called the locus coeruleus, which means "blue spot" (Poe et al., 2020). It is the essential home of the needed hormone norepinephrine, which impacts, among other things, arousal, blood pressure in times of stress, sleep patterns, mood, and memory (O'Donnell et al., 2012).

The orienting network is primarily involved with sensory aspects of the brain, and the way the senses serve to make sense of surroundings and recalibrate as needed (Posner et al., 2020). Think of the way we may either hyper focus or close our eyes in a moment of sensing danger. We may cover our ears in response to an off-putting noise. If we're looking for someone we know in a crowd, our whole body will start to zero in on them the moment we identify them. All the obvious or subtle ways we can utilize our senses to get our bearings relates to the orienting network.

The executing network includes task completion, threat assessing and response, self-regulation, conflict resolution, and voluntary response to input. Being the "executive," much of our day-to-day functioning can be traced back to the health of executing attention. Disruptions in the executing network correspond with a number of unwanted symptoms including hard-to-check fear, negative thoughts, recurring images, and addictive behaviors (Posner, 2020).

Improving Attention Networks

To return to the transportation analogy, availability is going to be different city to city. Some may have all three forms of transportation functioning smoothly and widely available. Others may have an outdated train system, or gridlocked streets at certain times of day. It's the same with individuals and attention. Each person will have different access to the three networks. Shaped by early years, experiences, brain health, and a myriad of other factors, we each have our own "transportation" systems with three networks that function differently.

Attention can't be reduced to focus, at least not for our purposes. Attention is about forming and strengthening helpful connections. It is about the relationship occurring between the self and the given context. It's the fact that there is a connection happening. The key is not whether you're good at focusing or whether you get distracted easily. Your attention is there, and there are connections happening between yourself and the various inputs within and around you. The resource is in the very real, universal ability to direct the connections being made. That ability is pivotal to mental health.

It can be easy to get stuck on how another city has better transportation, but chances are the networks available can get you where you need to go. You may have to supplement breakdowns in your attention with other skills. You may have to address some of the deterioration in your available systems. Good news: there are ways to improve those transportation networks, ways we can enhance attention.

Meditative practices support our attention networks (Esch & Schmidt, 2014). Support may be too tame a word for the transformative potential in some forms of meditation on attention. Meditation training can improve the quality of white matter in the brain, which translates to better self-regulation, with potentially a 10 percent improvement in attention functioning (Posner et al., 2019). While 10 percent may not seem like much, go back to the idea of city-transportation networks. Imagine 10 percent fewer cars in gridlock; imagine 10 percent more trains running on time; imagine a 10 percent increase in ferry departure times. It's not a small shift.

If any of these transportation networks were to boycott, the city could not function. In pursuit of improved mental wellness, we can't really afford to omit our attention networks. Thankfully, the ways of supporting them are accessible.

The Attention at our Disposal

For it to be a resource, the focus is specifically on the conscious aspects of attention. There is a whole lot of neural activity happening all the time as our systems respond to stimuli, and much of it happens imperceptibly or subconsciously (Latapie et al., 2022). The aim is the voluntary control of our attention, the parts of attention we can direct. In prioritizing the attention we have control over, we will mercilessly concentrate on what we can do and what makes it work for us.

Think of it like driving a car. As you go along, there is input in the form of other cars, traffic lights and signs, as well as the ever-changing landscape. Too often in life, we hold our attention more like a passenger in the car of our existence rather than as a driver able to give notice to the relevant aspects of our surroundings to navigate toward a desired destination. The goal is to direct attention to the pieces of input that matter, to orient to what's happening around us accurately, and to execute responses that steer our vessel in a way that accomplishes our goals. So it is with mental health. We aim to direct attention in order to align with our values, synchronizing incoming data with priorities, and in so doing alter experience and existence.

"The brain is capable of directing attention dynamically across extrapersonal space on the basis of expectations of where relevant events are likely to appear" (Coull and Nobre, 1998). In other words, in activities like driving a car, you have the ability to apply your mind to specific details, among the many, based on what is important to you. The same is true of daily living. Specific values guide the use of attention, both to recognize what may already be working and to scout out paths that lead where we want to go. We direct our attention by what we decide is important to us. In this we see two major, potentially life-altering points for focus. We can direct attention. We can decide what is relevant.

Directing Attention by Relevance

The brain's capacity to direct attention is a mechanism for mental wellness, a mechanism that humans initiate by setting relevance, values, and priority. Though it could take varying degrees of effort, the brain that signals my existence can also be selective about the connections I make between it and the world around me. The current state of mental health can change toward a specific, preferred quality.

Relevance is key. Attention is directed, prioritizing some data based on relevance or values (Anderson, 2016). So what determines what is relevant? Ultimately, you – if you're up for it. Are you conscious of what is important to you? Can you name the things that you want to characterize your life? If not, you may have attention that is being directed by a relevance prescribed by someone else. Maybe what your parents taught you. Maybe what your friends do. Maybe what you are pressured to believe is important. If you haven't named it for yourself, it's very likely that someone or something else is shaping how your attention is directed. When life has grown lackluster, it's possible that unclaimed attention is shaping our existence and experience. Reclaiming attention may be in order.

Directing attention is ownership of noticing. Relevance is ownership of values. Through attention, we triage input and make decisions for being *alert*, for how we *orient* ourselves to the world around us, and for how we *execute* our lives. We triage according to our values, the lens through which we place importance and priority. Attention is a resource we can direct purposefully or mindlessly. At times our attention is captivated by external forces, like when we hear a loud noise and all turn to look, or when fatigue is so strong that our mind is pulled away from the task at hand. Other times our attention is self-directed almost as a spotlight, like when we find our child on stage in the school program, or when reading the online medical records to see the test results.

To direct our attention mindfully is to identify and consider our values, and to direct connections between our existence and our experience accordingly. Without taking some ownership for how we can choose what we notice, connections are built by whatever is dominant. Without proactively identified values, we are either attending aimlessly, getting lucky occasionally, or allowing our attention to be hijacked by a force outside of ourselves. Here is our opportunity: direct attention through intentionally chosen relevance.

ATTENTION IN PRACTICE

With attention, as with many of these resources, each individual may have different capacities. Most important for change is the available and voluntary capacity. Let the other parts of attention be. If you are distractible, fine. If you are easily fixated, that's okay. The amount of attention in your control is the relevant and essential faculty for change.

In mental health we often say "what fires together, wires together" (Fishbane, 2007). By this we refer to the connections made between neurons, connections that are made stronger the more frequently they are utilized. So much of our mental processes happen involuntarily. And yet, we have the power to create, strengthen, and then utilize neural pathways. Attention can help us learn a skill to the point that it can be done without the same degree of active focus. After dedicating attention for a time to learning a new skill or way of being, we can move on. Then attention can be redirected to development of a new skill (Styles, 2006). In this way, the resource of attention becomes a catalyst for long-term integration of mental health practices. **We practice attention through mindfully directing relevant connections between existence and experience.**

Meditation Practice – A Guided Meditation Strengthening the Attention Networks

The provided guided meditation will lead you through use of the three attention networks. First is the alerting network, located in the brain stem and allows us to be conscious and aware. Second is the orienting network, which will be activated by a survey of the senses. Third is the executing network, located near the front of the brain and associated with conscious action (Posner et al., 2019). Go to kristaagler.com/book/keepinmind to listen to the provided audio or follow the accompanying prompts for a guided meditation strengthening the attention networks.

Reflection Practice – Identifying Values for Attention Relevance

Attention is allocated through a lens of values. In the field of psychology they're sometimes referred to as "pertinence values" (Styles, 2006). They are the forces that, because they matter more, guide our attention in specific directions. It's how we triage our attention in a given situation. Our values determine what's most important.

Identifying values allows us to take a proactive stance of attention that neurologically connects experience with existence on purpose. Be specific. Your lack of specificity is actively shaping every moment of your life. By specifically naming what is worthy of relevance in your life, attention will necessarily follow. Our identified values become the filter through which attention is alerted, oriented, and executed which influences mental wellness.

Respond to the following prompts with words or phrases, from which you will be able to draw out and identify specific values. From there, clarifying what each value means will strengthen the "pertinence." The act of externalizing responses (in writing, speaking, or typing) will strengthen those neural connections and be more useful to you. Avoid "just thinking" through the answers; our brains are too willing to take short cuts and keep the status quo. You can identify general values for life, and it may also be helpful to identify values for specific areas of life, such as marriage, work, creativity, parenting, spirituality, and so forth. Upon completing the exercise, you should have a list of five values with clarifying definitions. Of course you are not limited to five. Revisit as needed to maintain a list of values that is relevant and useful.

Table 2.1 Identifying Values for Attention Relevance

Prompts and Responses	
What do you want your life to be about?	
What do you want to be remembered for?	
Consider what makes you sad or angry. What about these things is important to you?	
How do you want to be for the people who are most important to you?	
What words describe the people you most want to be like?	
What are common features of times you felt proud, satisfied, or content?	
Identified Values Select five value words from the responses above and list them below. Identify what the value word means specifically and write one sentence of definition next to the value word.	
Value Word:	Definition:

Conscious Practice – Directing Attention According to Values

Identify one or two situations in life in which you'd like to see improvement. The first time you go through this practice, begin with a situation that is moderately troubling you. In learning the practice, keep it doable. Pushing yourself with the most challenging or disturbing troubles may be counter productive. Then, the work is to pair the difficult situation with an applicable value instead of the passive lenses that maladaptively shape daily living. By putting the situation and the value next to each other for consideration, attention is directed in such a way so as to shape the connection between existence and experience. A neurological change occurs with directed attention.

Shifting attention can apply to almost any life arena. For example, evaluating work through a lens of inconvenience may lead to discontent, while using a value lens of family or independence could strengthen mental connections between your work and your family or life goals. Similarly, looking at your marriage through a lens of criticism will bias attention toward faults, whereas a value lens of companionship will draw attention toward partnership. Considering friendships through the lens of loneliness will highlight experiences of disconnect perpetuating experiences of isolation, whereas a value lens of compassion, emphathy, or faith can foster connection even with distance.

Proceed through the following prompts. Reasonably and as you're ready, bring other areas of disruption in your life under the microscope and direct attention consistent with values.

Table 2.2 *Directing Attention According to Values*

Prompt	Situation 1	Situation 2
Identify a difficult situation or area of tension.		
Identify some desired values relevant to the situation.		
Consider the situation through that value lens. What do you notice?		
Where are aspects of the value present? Acknowledge the value in the situation.		
How could the value increase in the situation? Note aspects within your control.		

Lifestyle Practice – Anytime Redirection of Attention

To readily make use of the resource of attention in our daily lives, we need practices that are simple and easy to do every single day. In focusing on attention, you may find yourself noticing the many times your attention is drifting. It's normal and not to be avoided. The awareness itself becomes the opportunity. Any time you notice your attention is off the task at hand or on something not serving you in the moment, use that not as a time of frustration, but as the cue to direct your attention. You may direct your senses to what is immediately before you. You may make minor course corrections as you take inventory of your attention networks: alerting, orienting, executing. You may choose to recall a value that could be at play in the moment. You may simply do a brief interoception scan as you remain in motion. Any moment is an opportunity to direct attention.

One of the strongest aspects of attention is visual/spatial capacities (Coull and Nobre, 1998). In other words, attention will be more naturally drawn by what is prominent in the visual plane or what holds space in immediate physical surroundings. We can use this to our advantage. Using the values you identified describing your desired direction in life, create visual or spatial cues where they matter most. Consider placing words or images reflecting your values where they will enter your notice regularly. Alternatively, rearrange the physical location of items in a way that puts your values more central. If vision is unavailable or uncomfortable to you, use sound or tactile cues instead: an alarm on the phone, wind chimes near a door, or a small piece of fabric tied to a regularly used drawer pull or door knob. Intentionally shape your visual (or auditory or tactile) environment to work with your attention and desired values.

Make a list of five values and note the specific cue that will centralize awareness of the value in day-to-day functioning. Remember, these practices are meant to be simple so they can become part of our lives. Don't let their simplicity be mistaken for triviality.

IN SUMMARY

The Greek Stoic philosopher Epictetus said, "you become what you give your attention to" (Epictetus & Lebell, 1995). It follows that if you direct your attention, you can shape your experience and existence. The attention networks of alerting, orienting, and executing can be directed on purpose. Through identifying values, humans have the capacity to form attention toward our desired ends. Regular practice allows for improved mental health as both experience and existence reflect a life enriched by what is important to us.

REFERENCES

Anderson B. A. (2016). The attention habit: how reward learning shapes attentional selection. *Annals of the New York Academy of Sciences, 1369*(1), 24–39.

Coull, J. T. & Nobre, A. C. (1998). Where and when to pay attention: the neural systems for directing attention to spatial locations and to time intervals as revealed by both pet and fmri. *The Journal of Neuroscience: The Official Journal of the Society for Neuroscience, 18*(18), 7426–7435.

Epictetus, E. & Lebell, S. (1995). *The art of living: The classic manual on virtue, happiness, and effectiveness.* HarperOne.

Esch, T. & Schmidt, S. (2014). The neurobiology of meditation and mindfulness. In S. Schmidt & H. Walach (Eds.), *Meditation – Neuroscientifc Approaches and Philosophical Implications* (pp. 153–173). Springer.

Fishbane, M. D. K. (2007). Wired to connect: neuroscience, relationships, and therapy. *Family Process, 46*(3), 395–412.

Klink, P. C., Jentgens, P., & Lorteije, J. A. (2014). Priority maps explain the roles of value, attention, and salience in goal-oriented behavior. *The Journal of Neuroscience: The Official Journal of the Society for Neuroscience, 34*(42), 13867–13869.

Latapie, H., Kilic, O., Thórisson, K. R., Wang, P., & Hammer, P. (2022). Neurosymbolic systems of perception and cognition: The role of attention. *Frontiers in Psychology, 13*, Article 806397.

Lindsay, G.W. (2020). Attention in psychology, neuroscience, and machine learning. *Frontiers in Computational Neuroscience, 14*, 29.

O'Donnell, J., Zeppenfeld, D., McConnell, E., Pena, S., & Nedergaard, M. (2012). Norepinephrine: A neuromodulator that boosts the function of multiple cell types to optimize CNS performance. *Neurochemical Research, 37*(11), 2496–2512.

Poe, G. R., Foote, S., Eschenko, O., Johansen, J. P., Bouret, S., Aston-Jones, G., Harley, C. W., Manahan-Vaughan, D., Weinshenker, D., Valentino, R., Berridge, C., Chandler, D. J., Waterhouse, B., & Sara, S. J. (2020). Locus coeruleus: A new look at the blue spot. *Nature Reviews Neuroscience, 21*(11), 644–659.

Posner, M. I., Rothbart, M. K., & Ghassemzadeh, H. (2019). Restoring attention networks. *The Yale Journal of Biology and Medicine, 92*(1), 139–143.

Posner, M. I., Rothbart, M. K., & Ghassemzadeh, H. (2020). Developing attention in typical children related to disabilities. *Handbook of Clinical Neurology, 173*, 215–223.

Styles, E.A. (2006). *The psychology of attention.* Psychology Press.

Chapter 3

Will: A Resource of the Ability to Initiate Change

Though Wes had a gruff voice, his manners were soft. In his mid-fifties, he was timorous, but leathery. While in his twenties he had advanced in a narrow field, made lots of money, and found himself in circles of opulence beyond his maturity. He became involved with a woman who ran a nefarious network providing her with plenty of muscle. Within months, she had isolated him, orchestrated physical punishments for his attempts to leave, and eventually got control of his finances. For years, he was not permitted to leave the house to which he was designated. A learned helplessness settled in, and he grew accustomed to making no choices for himself.

His body began to deteriorate, and though the assumption was that this would be expected with the mistreatment he experienced, in reality cancer was spreading. When it became clear he may not survive, he was left outside of a hospital with no money and no identification. The social workers at the hospital provided some assistance, and for the next twenty years, he would stay on the move in between cancer treatments.

When he finally went to therapy, he was in remission, the cancer no longer detectable. He was homeless, tired, stalled. He was petrified of just about everything. Change began when a pivotal shift occurred. Helplessness took a hit when he was inspired to make an independent choice for himself. He wanted a dog. It was that simple. Through a government program, he secured housing and was to have his own place for the first time since his twenties. He saw a commercial with a dog in it, and that was it. He made a novel, internal decision, connecting a desire with intent. He formed a conscious, propelling choice. Like his hands finding the steering wheel again, it would be the first of many conscious, adaptive choices that would steer his life on a new course.

DOI: 10.4324/9781003521945-5

THE NATURE OF WILL

Imagine we are meeting at an agreed upon location. We are coming from different directions, and different distances. One of us has to drive through the city, navigating traffic along the way. The other, coming in from the country, faces long, winding roads. The weather for us is the same, perhaps sunny or perhaps a thunderstorm popping up. One of us is driving an old car, obtained for a good deal, nothing fancy but moving along. The other drives a newer make, temperature controlled, sound system immediately syncing. Perhaps a deer runs in front of one of us. And maybe the other has to pay at the tollbooth. Eventually we find ourselves at the appointed time and place.

Now, the majority of factors in our commute were different and largely out of either of our control. The ultimate destination wasn't deterred by those things. We could say that one of us may have had an easier or more enjoyable time, yet again, the ultimate destination isn't impacted even by that. We ended up at a desired destination because we both steered the car to get here.

Such sovereignty is the substance of will. As a captain steers a vessel amidst out-of-control elements, so will is on our side, endowing us with a rudder in waters beyond our authority. Identifying values may clarify where we want to go, but it is will that moves us there.

In the study of will from a mental health standpoint, a few terms give shape to the scope of what we're talking about. Defining those terms is a sound starting point. The term volition refers to the "series of decisions regarding whether to act, what action to perform and when to perform it" (Haggard, 2008). Self-efficacy is something we feel, the sense of having the ability to act. Agency is the experience that comes with actually carrying out an intended act (Haggard, 2017). Intention is a deliberately constructed statement aimed at shaping behavior. Will is the voluntary use and experience of all these concepts.

The concept of will, particularly within the field of psychology and neuroscience, is incredibly complex. For simplicity's sake, I have distilled a singular definition from all I've read as follows: Will is a faculty of control initiated on purpose. Will as a resource is not something that describes you, as if it's a personality trait. It is a capability every human has to govern the self. It's important that we see it as an ability or a skill to nurture, and not a quality we may or may not have.

The Faculty of Will

It is essential that we consider our will as a human faculty to set ourselves up to actually use it. And yet, even as we consider it as a faculty, from a brain perspective the will is not a force totally at your disposal. You don't have the capacity to independently direct every single thing you do every single moment of your life. Humans host a dynamic process for decision-making, of which a portion is within our sway (Schurger & Uithol, 2015). For mental wellness, it is important to not overestimate or underestimate our command of the will.

Will is a resource of faculty, shaping immediate and long-term influence on mental wellness. As we will come to find, we have a limited amount of control of what we do; yet the influence within that margin of autonomy is unique, potent, crucial, invaluable.

A key component of will as a resource is the degree of control within the ability. Now, there are wide disagreements about whether or not we as humans have free will (Smith, 2011). These discussions happen in the fields of psychology, neuroscience, behavior, law, philosophy, and religion. Do we really control ourselves, or are we the product of our genes, experiences, circumstances, and environment? And to what degree? Much of the research leads to the gray. Humans are not purely a predictable byproduct of the variables of our lives. Humans do not singlehandedly determine outcome by choice and grit alone. Between the extremes is our opportunity: to focus our energy on the control and influence available to us to shape our life and improve the world around us. Even if it's small, the role of volition matters a great deal.

The understanding and belief we hold of the will matters practically. If we don't think our efforts toward change make a difference, then we're hardly going to give it a fair attempt. It's worth asking yourself if you think your attempts matter. I believe they do. Will is an inherent mental skill that can be learned, strengthened, and applied.

Will isn't simply about wanting, though desire may be part of it. Will is distinguished from reaction and reflex by the ways it can go against impulse and move with forces like our values, motivations, and principles. The shift isn't from out of control to fully under control. The shift is from preoccupation, resignation, or even helplessness toward a deliberately intentioned will.

Healing Effect of Recovering Will

The health and use of will has direct mental health implications. Some may respond to a discussion about the will with little interest, depreciating the impact their choices can have. From my clinical observation, it seems the potential of the will to impact mental health goes undervalued. Often, the hardships that make exercising the will difficult leave a more robust harnessing of it untried.

In any struggle with mental health, or indeed in the wear and tear of daily living, a vital connection with our will can become strained. "I can't control my temper . . ." "I can't do simple things . . ." "I just can't stop . . . " Some of the most painful parts of mental illness come back to a disconnect from what is within our control. The experience of disrupted self-governing often results in painful symptoms or functional breakdown (Haggard, 2008).

Powerlessness is a key component of experiences that are considered traumatic (Kleber, 2019). A loss of control is typically present. As a therapist specializing in trauma treatment, one of the ways we work on trauma recovery is building up a connection to the ways we do have control, while also practicing acceptance of the things over which we do not have control (Boterhoven de Haan et al., 2021). It's an important distinction. In most experiences of trauma, it is true that there was an element that was beyond the control of the victim. It can create a generalized belief in an identity of powerlessness, thus inhibiting at best and damaging at worst the life of the victim even long after the trauma has ended. As we work to identify areas of control and mindful ways of initiating change, an important shift occurs in self-efficacy and agency.

A healthy connection to will is integral to mental wellness, perhaps especially after trauma, loss, or a prolonged plateau. Consider the following analogy from the natural world. When a caterpillar finds itself in a chrysalis, ready to begin its transformation into a butterfly, it starts to turn to goo (Gilman, 2018). It liquifies. It loses all sense of what it used to be, shape completely lost. Then it begins to rebuild, as if from scratch, taking on a previously unimaginable form. Even as it emerges, it's not yet ready to function. A fluid runs like streams through tiny veinlike threads woven into crumpled wads of tissue until smooth, flat, patterned wings stretch out (Osotsi et al., 2020). In trauma recovery, the reclamation of the will is the fluid filling lifeless wings until functioning is once again realized. Even if unrecognizable compared to the self prior to trauma, that filling equals a return to capacity and a recovery of volition.

The value and influence of a functional will extends beyond trauma recovery. It is essential to mental health, and what's more, it is a capacity available to everyone.

THE SCIENCE OF WILL

As neuroscientists study the brain, there is increasing evidence that we have less control of our behavior than we assume (Smith, 2011). Perhaps that is partly because we give attention to the parts of our "behaving" that are in our awareness, when a great deal of our movements, reactions, thoughts, words, and so forth are automatic, almost involuntary. Shockingly, it has been estimated that "only about five percent of our behavior is consciously controlled" (Baumeister et al., 1998). Consensus on the degree of control we have evades the fields of psychology, neuroscience, philosophy, and law. However, it is increasingly clear that it is less than we tend to think. Though it may be less in ratio than you'd like, the quality of its impact may be greater than what your current use of it indicates.

Will provides a mechanism for promoting significant change in our mental health with simple intention. To understand that mechanism and to be able to put it to use, we must be clear about what we mean with the word intention, and we must do business with the duality within the will, its passive and active qualities.

The Human Will as Two Systems

One perspective within the field of psychology breaks down the vast scope of human cognition and agency, or how we think and act, into two categories called System 1 and System 2. Now, most of the time if something complex is narrowed down to two options, it becomes reductionistic and some nuance is lost. The reason we do that is for clarity in what is admittedly complex. So there's some spectrum here and some interplay between the two systems. In fact, some propose a hybrid model due to the significance of the interplay between these systems and the apparent overlap between reason, intuition, reaction, and effortful thought (Bago & De Neys, 2020). Still, we will proceed with the simplified and widely accepted concept of two categories for the sake of understanding, and, therefore, the sake of usefulness.

In System 1 we have reflexive processes that are "fast, effortless, automatic and unconscious" (Schlosser, 2020). Immediate reaction, mental routines, intuition, and autopilot are some examples of functioning that would fall in this category. So when you brush your teeth, narrow your eyes in suspicion, complete any mundane part of your job, or have a strong reaction to a trauma trigger, System 1 is at work.

System 2 involves more conscious processes that are "slow, deliberate, controlled" (Schlosser, 2020). It includes processes like proactive problem-solving, reasoning, and restraint. You may find yourself using System 2 when you are learning a new skill, finding an alternative route to work due to unforeseen construction, or putting your best foot forward at a job interview.

You can see how most of the ways we think and act fall to varying degrees within these categories. Since we don't overtly control most of our daily movements and thought processes, it is then vital to accurately hone in on the thoughts we do direct and to distinguish the actions we do control.

The two categories have a way of working together. System 1 does the bulk of the work, helping us move about without conscious thought and conducting ourselves in a manner that has already been approved of previously. We don't have to relearn and redecide each thought and action. We can be on autopilot until System 2 intervenes either because a thought or action needs to be changed, or because a new thought or action is going to be initiated. Though System 2 can initiate novel activity on its own with conscious deliberation, it also has an override function to exert on System 1 when wanting to change a pattern already in place.

It's like driving a manual car. Most of the functioning of the car is automated, many different mechanisms working in tandem along with the almost unconscious monitoring of the gas pedal. And then you push the clutch in, shift, and continue in a different gear with conscious choice. So System 1 and System 2, though different, function with the other. They are also connected by a force that enables the practical application of the will. That force is "intention."

The Role of Intention in the Dual Functioning of the Will

In psychology and the study of human thinking, "intention" is a statement of a conscious decision to perform a behavior forged by conscious reasoning. Intention is not primarily about getting what you want, or reflecting on pleasant aspirations for your life. Do not confuse intention with sentiment. Intentions are definitive declarations about what you will do. Of course, these statements may be shaped by desire, but the things we want are fleeting, subject to change, and not always for good. Rather, intentions are best shaped by our stated values, the consciously reasoned priorities of ultimate importance. When shaped according to these higher principles, intentions clarify our thoughts and actions. The word "intentions" is sometimes used for ways we want to feel, but its real strength is in deliberate selection of what we will do to get where we want to go.

In the brain, there are a number of circuits involved in voluntary action. They all eventually merge at a crossroad called the primary motor cortex. This hub responds to a couple forms of input: voluntary input and what is called "stimulus-driven" input (Haggard, 2008). In other words, the primary motor cortex will respond to direct prompting from the self, or it will respond instinctively to external data. The facet of the primary motor cortex that follows voluntary input gives humans a quality of "stimulus-independence"; we have choice.

Just as human attention can be arrested by subconscious or external values, our intentions aren't always deliberate. It is possible to have unconscious intentions (Lavazza, 2016). Again, in approaching each resource to the extent that it can be utilized, the focus will remain on our capacity to form conscious intentions. Intentions are not a silver bullet as there is not a "single neural cause" to the will and decision-making (Schurger & Uithol, 2015). However, they are a required, basic component in choice, change, and improving mental health.

Intentions may include two different motivational dynamics in volition: decisions and degree of commitment (Rebar et al., 2018). So, what do you intend to do? And how serious are you about what you intend to do? It starts to become clear that intentions must be arrived at through careful consideration if they are to be useful. However, as simple statements of intention become clear, they activate both systems of the will.

Intentions are one way to reason and activate choice. They function differently between the two systems. The more overt presence is in System 2 where "intentional action" or "intentional agency" is the defining feature of controlled signaling. Intentions are also present in the more subconscious System 1 through "derivatively intentional" reflexes that have been shaped by intention. So there's a trickle-down effect, so to speak. What begins requiring System 2 conscious, deliberate problem-solving can eventually become System 1 routine (Schlosser, 2020).

Consider the process of teaching children almost any task or behavior: tying shoes, riding a bike, toileting, sharing, and so forth. At the outset, each element of the task is clearly defined and stated as a determined action step, or an "intention". Eventually, the intentions became routined and simple verbal reminders are enough. Hopefully in adulthood, these tasks that started out as foreign, complicated, and unnatural are all routine.

The rudimentary example of childhood simplifies the same pattern before us in pursuing change in our lives or mental wellness. Although it may be more complicated and the stakes may be higher, the major points are the same. Intentions are consciously formulated statements that activate System 2 of the will, eventually shaping System 1 autopilot. They are the mechanism by which we direct our course and reform mental health.

The Merit of Will Within Hardship

Though it may be different person-to-person, to be human comes with the ability to choose with purpose. Context may dictate the degree to which that faculty can be freely exercised. With limitations, perhaps with excruciating confines, a meager portion of will is useful, even vital.

You may be hard pressed, walls closing in. Perhaps your previous attempts at trying to change your circumstances have come up empty. Grief, trauma, and mental health struggles can significantly alter the experience of self-efficacy. It's one thing to talk about accessing the resource of will in hard times; it's another to live it. Many of the factors contributing to our mental health and well-being are beyond our control: genetic dispositions for mental illness; the degree of discord and brokenness in our nuclear family; our socioeconomic status with the associated limitations; experiences of trauma, loss of loved ones, injuries, and illness. The current state of objective reality, whatever the current experience, must be the starting point for recovering a sense of agency. Recentering the will transforms rather than dismisses hardship.

When we approach our mental health with an emphasis on our will, we begin shaping a mental health narrative of empowerment and self-determination. It's not about being self-made. It's about posture. Consider the difference between a swimmer's stroke and floating on your back. In still water both keep afloat. However, in troubled water the posture of propelling oneself with legs and arms working in tandem is preferred to passivity. In therapy, the work of noticing our control within hardship does not place false responsibility on victims; it restores agency, highlighting the ability and volition available to survive (Murray, 2015).

As a trauma therapist, much of my work has to do with what has happened to people in the past. Nevertheless, the method of approaching and processing the past over time shifts the perspective from not only what happened, to also the inherent qualities that contributed to survival, whether it be endurance, grit, strategy, faith, or simply holding on until it was over. A trauma survived tells a story beyond a wrong received and a chance survival. The will it takes to endure through the trauma to the present tells the story of a human ability to participate in changing the outcome.

WILL IN PRACTICE

What you can choose today, however small, is a more relevant reality than what happened then or is happening tomorrow, however large. The moments of the past had their say, impacting trajectory. The moments to come aren't ready to reveal themselves. Change comes through the narrow but sure intersection of now and the will. That is what's available to you.

We practice the resource of the will by consistently exercising volition with intention.

Meditation Practice – A Guided Meditation on Self-Efficacy and Agency

Practices of meditation produce changes in the brain that not only translate to more calm but they also increase the ability to observe our own preparations to act. Meditation can build more conscious involvement in decision-making as well as an increased capacity to act against problematic impulses (Jo et al., 2014). Go to kristaagler.com/book/keepinmind to listen to the provided audio or follow the accompanying prompts for a guided meditation on volition, self-efficacy, and agency.

Reflection Practice – Forming Intentions

Intentions draw from identified values and current context in the form of clear statements that influence thoughts, choices, and actions. The mental health practice of forming intentions involves a conscious decision to perform a behavior as a result of conscious reasoning (Schlosser, 2020). The goal is to clarify simple statements to guide future action. Values are pillars within intentions. It may also be helpful to reflect for a moment on where you would be in five years if your choices, actions, and life remained in alignment with those values. Use Table 3.1 and write down a sentence or two in reflection of your desired direction in the space provided. Then proceed with the exercise forming intentions. Examples provided are general, but in forming your intentions, be as specific as possible. Though only three prompts are provided, use them to create intentions for any areas of life that are important to you, that you encounter frequently, that challenge you, and that are difficult for you. By being thorough, more of your life and well-being will be subject to change through the influence of your intentions.

Conscious Practice – Working Within the Limits of Control with Intention

Acknowledging what is not within our control frees up internal reserves to do what is within our control. By acknowledging most of our behavior is automatic in the brain, we are freed up to narrow our efforts where we have influence. Intention is particularly useful within areas of restriction. Refer to Table 3.2. Begin by noting aspects of life beyond your control. Note: things that are in the past or in the future qualify as outside of your control. With

Table 3.1 Forming Intentions

Reflections on desired direction:		
Prompt	**Example**	**Intention**
Turn a value into an intention by naming a value and making a statement with (1) what you intend to do, and (2) why it is important to do it.	"I will work every day to build a life for my children that I did not have. I will provide for them, spend time with them, and tell them I love them every day."	
Apply a value to a current hardship to form an intention. Write a statement that names a valued action or posture that is possible in difficult times.	"I can be grateful even though this is a painful situation. I will express to one person each day how and why I appreciate them."	
Draw an intention from what is already going well. State how you can prioritize the actions or resources that already honor your values.	"I will continue to prioritize the supportive relationships I have. I will dedicate time and energy every week to the people I care about."	

compassion and resolve, accept that scenario as beyond your control at this time. Then, direct attention to where you do have influence, however small. Consciously write an intention statement identifying a value-consistent action that relates, however loosely, to that which is beyond control. You may find you have some agency and self-efficacy even within a situation that seems impossible.

Lifestyle Practice – Repetition to Strengthen Will

The concept of lifestyle carries more weight in the realization that the vast majority of our functioning happens on autopilot. Building routines that can then function independently are more important when they are given the respect of being our default mode. To make a behavior or mindset part of a lifestyle, it needs to be practiced often enough that the predictive functions of the brain can reliably take over. The practice isn't the end;

Table 3.2 Working within the Limits of Control with Intention

Situation Beyond Control	Intention
Example: The physical demands of work.	"I will care for my body by using the allotted breaks for eating food that helps my body. I will protect my sleep. I will familiarize myself with my rights as a worker related to breaks, paid time off, and related benefits. I will pursue promotion."
Example: Legal custody proceedings with former spouse.	"I will respond to my lawyer's request for information as quickly as possible. I will keep documentation in order. Most importantly, I will prioritize meaningful connection and laughter with my child when they are in my care."
Your situation:	Your intention:
Your situation:	Your intention:
Your situation:	Your intention:

it's the means to the ultimate desired direction. The point of practice is to utilize System 2 activity to the point of System 1 routine. Here, mindful repetition is helpful. Follow three steps to use repetition to strengthen the will within lifestyle:

First, practice your purposefully formed intentions daily through reading them or listening to recordings of them being read. Identify a specific plan of when and how to recite your intentions.

Second, regularly revisit where you want to see change in your life and mental health. Form an intention to that end and then add it to daily practice.

Third, at least weekly and preferably daily, take time to look over your stated intentions and mindfully direct attention to where you have thought or acted in accordance with those intentions. Notice the experience of agency, or what it feels like to do what you set out to do. Notice the experience of self-efficacy, or the growing awareness of the human capacity to act consciously.

IN SUMMARY

Will propels us from the stated intention to action, action to routine, and routine to change. Self-efficacy, agency, and volition play important parts in utilizing will as a resource. Intentions are mechanisms for purposeful, strategic change. As humans, most of our behavior is unconsciously executed; however, the portion of our behavior within our control can be crafted toward our desired ends. The two systems working together to form our actions allow for deliberate intervention if we so choose. Even within hardship, the human capacity for a degree of self-determination plays a dramatic role in healing and change. "Through their actions, humans . . . can transform the world around them, and also experience how they have transformed it" (Haggard, 2017). The resource of the will is ready for action.

REFERENCES

Bago, B., & De Neys, W. (2020). Advancing the specification of dual process models of higher cognition: A critical test of the hybrid model view. *Thinking & Reasoning, 26*(1), 1–30

Baumeister, R. F., Bratslavsky, E., Muraven, M., & Tice, D. M. (1998). Ego depletion: Is the active self a limited resource? *Journal of Personality and Social Psychology,* 74: 1252–1265.

Boterhoven de Haan, K. L., Lee, C. W., Correia, H., Menninga, S., Fassbinder, E., Köehne, S., & Arntz, A. (2021). Patient and therapist perspectives on treatment for adults with PTSD from childhood trauma. *Journal of Clinical Medicine, 10*(5), 954.

Gilman, C. (2018). Sleeping butterflies have spirited goo. *Journal of Experimental Biology. 221*(2).

Haggard, P. (2008). Human volition: towards a neuroscience of will. *Nature Reviews Neuroscience, 9*(12), 934–946.

Haggard, P. (2017). Sense of agency in the human brain. *Nature Reviews Neuroscience, 18*(4), 196–207.

Jo, H. G., Wittmann, M., Borghardt, T. L., Hinterberger, T., & Schmidt, S. (2014). First-person approaches in neuroscience of consciousness: brain dynamics correlate with the intention to act. *Consciousness and Cognition, 26,* 105–116.

Kleber, R. J. (2019). Trauma and public mental health: a focused review. *Frontiers in Psychiatry, 10*(June).

Lavazza, A. (2016). Free will and neuroscience: from explaining freedom away to new ways of operationalizing and measuring it. *Frontiers in Human Neuroscience, 10,* Article 197548.

Murray, M. (2015). Narrative psychology. *Qualitative psychology: A practical guide to research methods,* 85–107.

Osotsi, M. I., Zhang, W., Zada, I., Gu, J., Liu, Q., & Zhang, D. (2020). Butterfly wing architectures inspire sensor and energy applications. *National Science Review, 8*(3), Article nwaa107.

Rebar, A. L., Dimmock, J. A., Rhodes, R. E., & Jackson, B. (2018). A daily diary approach to investigate the effect of ego depletion on intentions and next day behavior. *Psychology of Sport and Exercise, 39,* 38–44.

Schlosser, M. (2020). Dual-System Theory and the Role of Consciousness in Intentional Action. In B. Feltz, M. Missal, & A. Sims (Eds.), *Free Will, Causality, and Neuroscience* (Vol. 338, pp. 35–56).

Schurger, A., & Uithol, S. (2015). Nowhere and everywhere: The causal origin of voluntary action. *Review of Philosophy and Psychology, 6*(4), 761–778.

Smith, K. (2011). Neuroscience vs philosophy: taking aim at free will. *Nature, 477*(7362), 23–5.

Chapter 4

Thought: A Resource of Voluntary Mental Events

At forty-five years old, Nina would describe herself as timid and agreeable. However, behind the closed doors of therapy, she expressed strongly held opinions and a fierce desire to advocate for others. There were two competing portraits. In her fifteen years of marriage, she quietly witnessed her husband's mistreatment of herself and eventually their children. She had an awareness of her tendency to sidestep his anger and to teach the kids how to avoid upsetting him. At the beginning of their relationship, she had thought they were a good match as both of their families celebrated how they balanced each other, her quiet stability rounding out his passion. She was told how she had been the same for her father: a sweet, agreeable girl that went along with her rough old man.

Watching her children step into the same role she had assumed most of her life changed her perspective. A role she previously accepted no longer seemed like balance but rather like approving inappropriate behavior. She thought she was timid, and she thought that was a good thing. She thought she was responsible for the abusive behavior of those around her. And she thought there was no way the situation could change. Until, eventually these thoughts became unacceptable to think about her children.

Many of these thoughts had been shaped by her upbringing and more recent trauma. For the sake of her children, she began challenging these thoughts and considering other perspectives. Nina spoke over her children the kind truths she had not heard as a child, and found it began to alter her own story. She thought of herself differently when she discovered that the limiting factor was her own perception of herself as timid and stuck, and that the remedy was a more thoroughgoing honesty. The truth she spoke to her children and then to herself, she eventually told to her

DOI: 10.4324/9781003521945-6

husband who himself had been shaped by unfit words and abusive upbringing. The slow dismantling of thoughts of who they were and how they had to be left room for an entirely new construction of their family.

THE NATURE OF THOUGHT

As I've considered how to convey the role of thought as part of a mental health lifestyle, it has been tempting to not include it. The world of the mind, the complexity of thought, and the uniqueness of each individual's thought patterns are vast, far beyond the scope of a single chapter. I know I can't do the topic justice. However, the potency of thought and how it actively improves or deteriorates mental health means it can't be neglected. The reality of hard circumstances can be daunting, and the idea that thought change would be helpful can seem flimsy. Still, the damage done by those hard circumstances means we don't have the luxury of remaining passive in our thinking. Even with the potential discomfort of wrangling troublesome thought patterns, we cannot forfeit the opportunity for whole-life impact that thought change brings. **Thought is the resource of voluntary mental events by which we mold our experience and functioning.**

With the goal of utilizing available resources for improving mental wellness, thought is an essential. For it to be of help to you and to me in practical living, we will need to be precise in our definition of and focus on "thought." I will not exhaustively explain how thoughts work or the neuroscience behind them. I will, however, define a small sector of thought, particularly the parts that can be addressed to bring relief, redirection, and change.

Consider thoughts like the rain. Imagine looking out your window during a storm. It comes down in broad sheets, but as you look closer you notice how water touches everything and begins to gather in cracks in the road and along the curb. Perhaps on the window, you can distinguish a single drop trailing down the glass. Only some of the rain falls on your roof, collected by the gutter, and then channeled through downspout, perhaps into a rain barrel from which the water could be used for specific purposes. Similarly, thoughts fall en masse and only a portion are conscious, and an even smaller fraction of those can be gathered and utilized. The vast majority of our cognition, or thinking, is involuntary: outside of our control and sprouting spontaneously (Krans et al., 2015). And yet, some of our thoughts are voluntary: chosen, highlighted, encouraged (Kelly & Setman, 2020). In the forthcoming discussion on thought, we are purposely ignoring a world of rain and focusing on the drops coming down the drainpipe. The rain at large, or the force of our unbidden thoughts, can cause us great concern. However, it is the smaller portion of thoughts that can be collected, channeled, and applied which are of utmost importance, because that is the portion we can put to good use.

Prioritizing Voluntary Thought

The brain and our capacity for thinking is dizzyingly complex. Our scope of thought will be unapologetically narrow. When considering thought as a resource, we are talking about the slim margin of it within our awareness and within our voluntary influence, the thoughts we can control or initiate.

Involuntary thoughts are the vast majority and are the ones we don't control. Involuntary thoughts can be troubling to people, perpetuating negativity, reminding of past trauma, or replaying narratives that keep us from living fully (Shapiro, 2012). Although their effect is real and important, the dynamic of involuntary thoughts being outside of our control invites us to leave them alone, for now, and to focus instead on the phenomenon of voluntary thoughts, where change is possible.

Mental Events, Reality, and Perception

For the purpose of practical mental health, a thought can be defined as a voluntary or involuntary mental event occurring in the brain and experienced in the mind. It can be liberating to begin viewing thoughts as mental events as opposed to incidents of reality. Mental events can cause disruption, elation, or pain (Shapiro, 2012), and yet they remain occurrences within the mind. Distinguishing between a response to a mental event and to an incident of reality is an important skill. In my clinical observation, I often observe mental events initiating a response as if the thought were an incident of reality. A thought of future trouble or of current misunderstanding can initiate physiological discomfort and even miscalculated decision-making. Alternatively, confining our reality to what is objective and observing mental events for what they are can ease and simplify the burden of response. The incident of reality is the unarguable fact of the matter, such as your partner walking in the door after work and not saying much. The mental event is initiated in part by reality and in part by perception, such as the thought "he must be upset with me because he is quiet." Responding to the latter may or may not be called for, and separating the two allows us to consciously choose a response more intentionally. Our thoughts and reality understandably weave together: the pending test results and the fear of the result, news of potential layoffs and the threat of lost income, or the news headline and the subsequent anxiety. They may come hand in hand, but they can be addressed independently. Reality monitoring is the process responsible in part for this distinction (Simons et al., 2017).

Reality monitoring is also the process through which we hold our perception accountable (Simons et al., 2017). As we take in an experience through our senses, we make sense of it through our previous experiences. It is the representation of reality the mind holds based on the interplay between mental events and incidents of reality. Reality is verifiable to varying degrees, and, "as science and common sense assume, there is one public all-embracing physical space in which physical objects are" (Russell, 2012). Perception must be accurate to a degree to be useful; inaccurate perceptions are problematic. Reliable perceptions are referred to as veridical perceptions, and one way these are checked is through the senses (Hoffman et al., 2015). The human mind experiences reality as a verifiable perception, shaped through the organization of the senses, the learned pattern of past experiences, and our cognitions or mental events. Our cognitions, our senses, and specifically how we manage them both influence our perception. It doesn't change reality, but it does influence our understanding of the world and our experience of it. Well-maintained senses and cognitions make for a better functioning mental health.

Perception of thoughts, voluntary or involuntary, occurs in the mind, which we've distinguished from the brain. Remember the brain is a specific organ in your body that functions mechanistically. The mind is more abstract, and so it may help to refresh what we're talking about. The mind is the element in a person by which perception, organization, and mental activity exists. It is present in every person. The mind, for the sake of our conversation, is not about your aptitude or about mental capacity. It is about the very present element within each human through which we engage in the act of living. It is a necessary gift that much of it functions without our control or notice, and it is equally a wonder that part of it functions with our influence. It is a good thing that most of our thoughts are automatic, which is why we are spared recreating our perception of reality every time we step out our front door. The brain is incredibly adept at painting the picture. It is also good that we hold the power of voluntary thought, maintaining the capacity to improve our perception. We can correct or optimize perception in order to better serve mental wellness.

It is worth noting: the disruption of trauma can sometimes blur the line differentiating the experience of a mental event and incidents of reality. It goes beyond perception. When an experience of trauma is maladaptively stored in the brain, one of the reasons why it is so disruptive is that the memory connects to parts of the brain both of the past and of the present-tense alarm system. The mental event of the memory lights up with the sensory perception centers connected to actual reality (Shapiro, 2012). The line between a mental event and an incident of reality is blurred at a brain level. As trauma therapists, we're referencing this neurological reality when we use the word "trigger," which stands in contrast to its common use today that seems to apply to anytime a person experiences an uncomfortable emotion, memory, or offense. There are mental events we can adjust if we choose; and there are mental events blurred at a brain level with sensory experiences of an incident of reality. The latter can also be mended, but it's worth noting that they are very different.

A moment of reality is unchanged by our momentary perception, but perception alters our experience and then how we live based on that experience (Drigas & Mitsea, 2020). The human system can adaptively relate to reality through improved perception, and the careful selection of cognitions can change our experience of even the unchangeable aspects of reality. What is required is strategic and purposeful stewardship of mental events. We move now to reliable, research-based ways of doing just that.

THE SCIENCE OF THOUGHT

There are a variety of methods of addressing thoughts. Cognitive Behavioral Therapy (CBT) is a therapeutic intervention focused on the mental health improvements that come from cognitive change. It is an approach that boasts more positive response rates than comparative treatments and stands on a strong evidence-base foundation (Hofmann et al., 2012). Although treatment of cognitions is only one part of a holistic approach to mental wellness, it is nevertheless an essential part. **Thought provides the opportunity to select mental content that can favorably impact how we think, feel, and live.**

We can target sustainable thought change by devoting effort to a few forms of voluntary thought: directed thought, narratives, and data input. The science here is not on the brain or the complexity of how thoughts work; it is the proven methods of improving symptoms through harnessing thought.

Directed Thought

There is a cascade of involuntary thoughts beyond our control that can be uncomfortable, disruptive, and even painful. However, the landscape of the mind is not shaped entirely by involuntary thoughts (Schlosser, 2020). We can use active thoughts to interrupt and redirect the vast amount of ongoing, passive thoughts. It is a continual dance between the involuntary and the voluntary. It is an exchange of ideas going on perpetually. Involuntary thoughts stream and voluntary thoughts intervene. We can consciously direct voluntary thoughts to respond to the mass of involuntary thoughts that arise (Wells, 2019).

As humans, we reserve the ability to decide whether or not we permit certain thoughts to go unchallenged. It's easier said than done, but it is possible. We have a capacity for what's called "top-down" controlled influence of our patterns. Our use of "dynamic control" and responsiveness can directly impact our mental wellness, even though it is outweighed by the quantity of our passive thinking (Wells, 2019). Insofar as we are resigned to our involuntary thoughts, we are impacted by the people and experiences that shape them. In this case, thoughts are controlled by external factors. The alternative is to direct thoughts within our control – changing current mental events and shaping future involuntary thoughts.

Directed thought uses attention and will to initiate a mental event consistent with values and desired direction. The potential here is significant: even in the face of long-held thought patterns or troubling, disruptive "self-talk," the mind has the capacity to go a different direction. Neuroimaging technology has shown how cognitive practices of directing thoughts, or what is also called selective perception, can bring long-term neurobiological change (Jokić-Begić, 2010). Cognitive activity, both at a level of observed thoughts and also at a neurological level, can be improved through sustained use of simple, directed thought.

Our minds are constantly recalibrating, taking in our surroundings or the information available and reorienting accordingly (Sara & Bouret, 2012). When we consciously interrupt thinking that is not helpful or add an intentional thought, our mind reorients with the added information. When we respond with voluntary thoughts that are more helpful, more intentional, and more in line with our values, then our minds recalibrate to that effect. It's the often-used analogy of the trajectory of a flight: I may alter course by only one degree, and in a few moments time the final destination is miles different. Small changes matter.

Narratives

If you were to turn on the TV and flip back and forth between a few different news channels, you will likely catch the same story told in a variety of ways. You may notice that although the details of date and time and number may be similar, you will hear very different stories of the same event. Those different stories affect emotions, choices, mindsets, relationships, and so forth. The stories couching the details are themselves a powerful influence.

The human brain similarly organizes details of thought and mental activity within stories, or what are often called "narratives." In the mind, the same set of details can be organized in a variety of narrative patterns, woven with additionally chosen thoughts. Even when situations are unchangeable, the narrative can produce various effects because they influence brain activity patterns (Song et al., 2021).

The narratives we choose may or may not be consistent with our values or even with reason. The narratives we accept and repeat affect our response, and affect our mental wellness. Functional neuroimaging reveals that as the brain integrates narratives, brain states are affected (Song, et al., 2021). With voluntary thought, we choose which narratives we accept, which narratives we repeat, and which narratives we choose to tell ourselves given the fixed details of our lives. The process integrates the pieces of information, altering the brain in a way that ripples into our emotions, responses, choices, and future thinking.

To optimize the process, a well regulated brain will construct and integrate narratives in a more adaptive way. Neuroscience-informed psychotherapy indicates that narrative approaches to thought change are best applied after emotional and physical regulation (Takizawa et al., 2022). Just as senses are part of our perception, they can also be mindfully utilized to increase regulation that in turn improves the brain's use of narratives.

With regulation, we need to tell better, holistically honest stories. Take the narratives of mental health as an example. Many clinicians and laypeople alike, in attempts to address problems and obstacles to mental health, settle into a narrative that is problem-centric, emphasizing what may be wrong. The imbalance may cause identity to be formed by what's happened to a person and how they feel about it. Though acknowledging a problem is essential and cultivating environments that encourage openness are also needed, there is a part of the story to be told that goes beyond the problem.

In therapy, one proposed solution to such a lopsided tendency is a method called a "double-storied" approach, which is an avenue of treatment inviting people to tell the full story, both the hardship and the strength, the pain and the resilience (Peterson, 2021). They are equally true, and should be equally told. The beautiful thing about approaching life in a "double-storied" way is that often the hopeful, capable, and surviving aspects of the story are already present; they only require attention and telling.

In my clinical observation, as every single one of my trauma clients have told me the stories of what they've been through, there is evidence of their resilience. The good may be hard to see as it is overshadowed by the darkness of the suffering. It's understandable. Nevertheless, the reward of digging through the story in order to clearly state the good, the virtue, the strength, and the genius can be a watershed moment. It doesn't cancel out the impact of the trauma, but it does make the story-to-come quite different. In not ignoring the pain, the power of narratives takes the unchangeable details and doesn't stop there: it proceeds to simply tell the full story. As the double-storied narrative is integrated, brain patterns change and so does the quality of life. Without having to change circumstances, we change the story, the brain, and mental health.

Data Input

The content of our thoughts is a sizable factor in our well-being (Segerstrom et al., 2003). Some thoughts may be externally generated, initiated by the words and actions of others, by life experiences, or by environment. Many of our thoughts are also self-generated (Andrews-Hanna et al., 2013). Data input refers to our self-generated thoughts as well as the role we have in monitoring externally generated thought content.

Content consumption, particularly of a violent or alarming nature, not only impacts emotions and state but also influences future thinking, particularly in the form of intrusive thoughts (Holman et al., 2020). What we listen to, what we read, who we are around, what we watch, and where we go goes beyond affecting the brain-body system in the moment and becomes part of the available pool of content from which we draw future thoughts, motivation, emotions, and behavior (Tiggemann & Anderberg, 2020). The data digested in a day becomes part of the human system long after the moment of consumption. Dedication to mental wellness requires conscious management of the thought content we seek and allow.

We may be fairly rigid about who we allow in our homes. We can be vigilant about not eating certain kinds of food. Yet, human culture at large seems woefully hands off about gatekeeping the content of thoughts. What data you consume today is not simply here today and gone tomorrow. It has potential to become part of the mental reserves from which you draw your reflexive behavior and cognition. Beyond the importance of the quality of thought content, the act itself of monitoring data is a buildable skill. The thought control exercised in monitoring data input is beneficial not just because we can limit negative content and seek out beneficial content; it will also be reflected in cognitive patterns from which we live functionally. We develop the skill of more strategic thinking and useful discernment for the future to come (Segerstrom et al., 2003).

One study, seeking to identify the types of content most beneficial to well-being, found that the most adaptive data was "positive, less personally significant, and more specific" (Andrews-Hanna et al., 2013). First, positive content would be the data that aligns with what benefits the system, what serves the surrounding environment, and what coincides with our values. Positive versus negative isn't primarily about your preferences or mine; it's about what helps the brain-body system rather than harming it. Second, perspective that doesn't singularly prioritize the self but also considers others is beneficial to well-being. A hyperfocus on oneself causes various levels of psychological disruption. Seeing others to be as significant as the self is helpful. Third, mindful specificity works against the negative bias that can take over with general views of life. Consider the often used phrase, "I'm really busy." As a generality, it can foster a negative sense of being. Reflection on the specifics that amount to being busy can call to mind pleasant tasks, valued people, challenges met, and so forth. Encouraging specific data in thought content is more beneficial to well-being than generalities.

Data input is mental health ground not to be forfeited. Curate thoughts to produce life change. Conscious consumption of information is a holistic, available intervention. The resolute filtering of incoming data paves cognitive patterns for ongoing benefit.

THOUGHT IN PRACTICE

Perhaps you sense your mind is a strength, vibrant and alert. Or, perhaps you feel your mind is unreliable due to injury, illness, or inability. In any case, there is a portion of your mind that responds to your direction. Intentional application of thought is a powerful resource, available in some measure to all. Carefully chosen voluntary thoughts send ripples through the mind, body, emotions, behavior, and lifestyle. **We practice thought by selecting and directing mental events, elevating brain patterns.**

Meditation Practice – A Guided Meditation on Thought Observation

With the tendency to identify ourselves with our thoughts, a first step to cognitive change is the practice of observing thoughts. Almost like stepping off the stage and taking a seat, we can notice the theater of our life and begin observing mental events, facts of reality, input from the senses, and so forth. The first step in channeling the resource of thought is to become an observer of our thoughts as mental events. Go to kristaagler.com/book/keepinmind to listen to the provided audio or follow the accompanying prompts for a guided meditation on thought observation.

Reflection Practice – Creating Double-Storied Narratives

Narratives are like a mental map of how we orient ourselves. They are the way we characterize the problems, the goals, and the settings of our life. Whether we own it or not, these stories directly inform our mental wellness by altering brain states. The practice in Table 4.1 will assist in using the resource of thought to more beneficially shape our narratives of the past and present. The focus here is careful honesty that neglects neither the favorable or the trying. Remember, changes in narratives are strongest when we start from a place of regulation. Slowly, settle into a posture to take time. Exhale fully. Complete the following exercise. Repeat the work of constructing new narratives with as many areas of life that require reframing.

Conscious Practice – Directing Thoughts

There is an ongoing internal dialogue between involuntary and voluntary thoughts. Directing thoughts is our opportunity to change the conversation. By tuning into unhelpful involuntary thoughts, we can then purposefully respond with a directed thought. In so doing, we exert some "top-down" influence – shifting perception, experience, and behavior.

In Table 4.2, the goal is to begin by focusing on three problematic thoughts. To track down a problematic thought, begin with areas of life with dysfunction or discomfort. Consider a statement that sums up your mindset about that part of life. Look for ways in which that mental event is problematic: Is it inaccurate? Is it unnecessarily negative? Does it run counter to your values? Then, respond deliberately to each. Form directed thoughts that are more accurate, more helpful, and more in-line with what matters most to you.

Lifestyle Practice – Routine Thought Filter

How we think about how we think matters. It impacts everything. "Metacognition (thinking about thinking) refers to the structures, content, and processes involved in the monitoring, appraisal, and control of cognition" (Wells, 2019). To step into this thinking-about-thinking is to become active navigators toward mental wellness. Beyond formal practices, our daily life and indeed our moment by moment mental wanderings become available opportunities to course-correct. With identified values, intentions, and some clarity on how to direct thoughts, rewrite narratives, and input desired data, that course correction becomes effective.

Table 4.1 Creating Double-Storied Narratives

<table>
<tr><th>Past Prompt</th><th>Response</th></tr>
<tr><td>Describe in 3–5 words the struggles of your life up to now.</td><td></td></tr>
<tr><td>Describe in 3–5 words the strengths you have demonstrated during your life.</td><td></td></tr>
<tr><td colspan="2">Construct a double-storied narrative pairing struggle with strength. Fill in the blanks below.

Example: “My life has been characterized both by loss and celebration, by insecurity and endurance, by loneliness and creativity.”</td></tr>
<tr><td colspan="2">Fill in:

“My life has been characterized both by__________ and __________,

by__________ and __________, by __________ and __________.”</td></tr>
<tr><th>Present Prompt</th><th>Response</th></tr>
<tr><td>Identify a current challenge or struggle.</td><td></td></tr>
<tr><td>Identify helpful traits of your personality or ability.

Identify sources of support in your life.</td><td></td></tr>
<tr><td colspan="2">Construct a double-storied narrative pairing challenge with sources of help and support. Fill in the blanks below.

Examples: “Even though I lost my job, I am able to respond with grit.”

“Even though my pain is flaring today, I have a partner and a bed to support me.”</td></tr>
<tr><td colspan="2">Fill in:

“Even though ____________________, I am ____________________.”

“Even though ____________________, I have ____________________ to support me.”</td></tr>
</table>

Table 4.2 *Directing Thoughts*

Directions: *In the left-hand column, write down three problematic thoughts in the form of a sentence. Then, in the right-hand column, respond with a thought that is more accurate, helpful, and aligned with your values.*	
Problematic Thought	**Directed Thought**
Example: "I hate uncertainty. Not knowing what's going on causes me anxiety."	Example: "Uncertainty is part of life, and I have options for how to respond. I can rely on my values of hard work and friendship to be more prepared for uncertain situations. There are things within my control to calm my nervous system even in uncertainty."

Learning to calibrate our thoughts is like learning to drive a car. At the outset, it requires paying attention and purposeful movements. Over time, and fairly quickly, what felt like a sizable task becomes automated and routine. You steer primarily through constant, imperceptible adjustments. So it can be with thought.

As you go about life, regularly check in with your thoughts. Do so in the normal rhythm and motion of your life, yet do so directly, with purpose. Perhaps, use the questions in Table 4.3 as a filter.

In other words: You are telling the story; tell it all. You shape your perception; shape it on purpose. You are a gatekeeper of mental content; be selective.

Table 4.3 *Routine Thought Filter*

Today, how can I describe life events in a way that is more double-storied than problem-centric?
Today, how can I redirect thoughts to improve my experience of circumstances?
Today, how can I filter problematic thoughts and respond to them with directed thoughts?

IN SUMMARY

More than an internal running commentary, thoughts are potent data pieces that, in their right standing, can be directed to change brain patterns. Our experience of existence is shaped by perception, which is comprised of phenomena including our mental events, facts of reality, and input from the senses. By taking advantage of the voluntary thoughts within our control, we can directly improve perception, experience, neural circuitry, mood, mental state, and behavior.

The human relationship to thought is not meant to be one of passivity, as if thoughts mastermind a condition to which we are subject. We do not serve our thoughts, but rather, they are available to serve us as a resource for mental wellness. The mental events populating our minds are open to our orchestrating – if we are willing to conduct.

REFERENCES

Andrews-Hanna, J. R., Kaiser, R. H., Turner, A. E., Reineberg, A. E., Godinez, D., Dimidjian, S., & Banich, M. T. (2013). A penny for your thoughts: Dimensions of self-generated thought content and relationships with individual differences in emotional wellbeing. *Frontiers in Psychology, 4,* 900.

Drigas, A., & Mitsea, E. (2020). The 8 pillars of metacognition. *International Journal of Emerging Technologies in Learning, 15*(21), 162–178.

Hoffman, D. D., Singh, M., & Prakash, C. (2015). The interface theory of perception. *Psychonomic Bulletin & Review, 22,* 1480–1506.

Hofmann, S. G., Asnaani, A., Vonk, I. J., Sawyer, A. T., & Fang, A. (2012). The Efficacy of Cognitive Behavioral Therapy: A Review of Meta-analyses. *Cognitive Therapy and Research, 36*(5), 427–440.

Holman, E. A., Garfin, D. R., Lubens, P., & Silver, R. C. (2020). Media exposure to collective trauma, mental health, and functioning: Does it matter what you see? *Clinical Psychological Science, 8*(1), 111–124.

Jokić-Begić, N. (2010). Cognitive-behavioral therapy and neuroscience: Towards closer integration. *Psihologijske teme, 19*(2), 235–254.

Kelly, D., & Setman, S. (2020). The psychology of normative cogniation. In E. N. Zalta (Ed.), *The Stanford Encyclopedia of Philosophy* (Spring 2021 ed.). Stanford University.

Krans, J., de Bree, J., & Moulds, M. L. (2015). Involuntary cognitions in everyday life: Exploration of type, quality, content, and function. *Frontiers in Psychiatry, 6*(7).

Peterson, J. (2021). Moving beyond the single story: Using a double-storied assessment tool in narrative practice. Dulwich Centre.

Russell, B. (1912). *The problems of philosophy.* Oxford University Press.

Sara, S. J., & Bouret, S. (2012). Orienting and reorienting: The locus coeruleus mediates cognition through arousal. *Neuron, 76*(1), 130–141.

Schlosser, M. (2020). Dual-System Theory and the Role of Consciousness in Intentional Action. In B. Feltz, M. Missal, & A. Sims (Eds.), *Free Will, Causality, and Neuroscience* (Vol. 338, pp. 35–56).

Segerstrom, S. C., Stanton, A. L., Alden, L. E., & Shortridge, B. E. (2003). A multidimensional structure for repetitive thought: what's on your mind, and how, and how much? *Journal of Personality and Social Psychology, 85*(5), 909.

Shapiro, F. (2012). *Getting past your past: Take control of your life with self-help techniques from EMDR therapy.* Rodale.

Simons, J. S., Garrison, J. R., & Johnson, M. K. (2017). Brain mechanisms of reality monitoring. *Trends in Cognitive Sciences, 21*(6), 462–473.

Song, H., Park, B. Y., Park, H., & Shim, W. M. (2021). Cognitive and Neural State Dynamics of Narrative Comprehension. *The Journal of Neuroscience: The Official Journal of the Society for Neuroscience, 41*(43), 8972–8990.

Takizawa, Y., Murray, J., Bambling, M., Matsumoto, Y., Ishimoto, Y., Yamane, T., & Edirippulige, S. (2022). Integration of clinical neuroscience into psychotherapy: A narrative review of neuroscience-informed psychotherapy models for the treatment of depression and anxiety disorders. *Psychotherapy and Counselling Journal of Australia, 10*(1).

Tiggemann, M., & Anderberg, I. (2020). Social media is not real: the effect of "instagram vs reality" images on women's social comparison and body image. *New Media & Society, 22*(12), 2183–2199.

Wells, A. (2019). Breaking the cybernetic code: understanding and treating the human metacognitive control system to enhance mental health. *Frontiers in Psychology, 10,* 2621–2621.

Chapter 5

Span: A Resource of Potential and Limits

Jones would say he led a simple life. He went to the office from eight to five, went home, and in the evenings and on the weekends he answered emails and tied up loose ends. He spent time with his kids, took care of house projects, volunteered cleaning at his church, went to obligatory social functions, drove his children to and from sporting events and sleepovers, drove the few hours to visit his aging parents every other week, occasionally watched a basketball game with friends from high school, and managed his diabetes. And he would try to spend time with his wife. And exercise when he could. A simple life.

A slow, progressive onset of symptoms began to complicate matters. It started with bouts of shortness of breath and his heart racing. Doctors assured him that he was healthy. Next, his sleep became disrupted even though he felt exhausted all the time. Eventually, getting ready for work or even opening up his computer brought with it a sense of dread. He lost enjoyment in the few activities that used to bring him happiness, and he became harsh with his family yet hated himself for it. His thoughts became dark and despairing. He looked at his life and saw nothing unusual. He would explain how he "just folded up and waited for things to get better." Until, one day his wife said enough was enough, and something needed to change.

Jones went to therapy, "because she made me," trying to keep his wife from going through with the separation. He suspected the unignorable depressive and anxiety symptoms were related to his diabetes and the doctor just didn't get it. As if to demonstrate how his diabetes was the only possible threat, he explained his "simple life." He was surprised when the therapist observed, "if I took a healthy, happy brain and put it in your

DOI: 10.4324/9781003521945-7

lifestyle and gave it three weeks, it would experience exactly what you're experiencing."

Together, they unpacked the pile of commitments he tried to juggle, acknowledged limits, and prioritized the necessary and the beneficial. He quit compulsory social events, reserving leisure time for date nights with his wife and watching basketball with friends. He traded the "chore of working out" for a biweekly open gym, playing basketball with the same friends and investing more in those relationships. As a family, they reduced their extracurricular commitments by half and made the regular trips to care for grandma and grandpa together. Jones found himself breathing easier, looking forward to the week ahead, and able to appreciate the people and work in his life. He would later express, "I didn't realize the slow death I was in until it was almost too late".

THE NATURE OF SPAN

Span refers to one's extent or reach. It connotes both expanse and boundary. The fullness and the edge. In reference to the holistic person, span marks where we reach full potential while also respecting limits. It includes the full, internal extent of your mental person, including personality, IQ, and faculties. It includes the full, external extent of your physical person, height, weight, physical capacity, and body rhythms. And it includes the full, communal extent of your relational person: how you talk with others, touch them, rely on them, and are available to them. Within that extent is your potential, a sweet spot for mental wellness where the human brain-body system benefits from energizing activity and from healthy balance. **Span is the resource of mental flourishing that comes with reaching potential and honoring limits.**

Considering Limits

You have an extent, meaning, there is a place in which you are, and then there is a place where you are not. There's a limit. Some limits are easier to admit than others. It may be easy to admit the ways your height limits certain athletic endeavors; it may be more difficult to say you don't have time or energy for a task that a friend wants you to do.

There is an aspect of culture that seeks to push limits, to go beyond them, and in many ways we have exceeded what was previously thought to be humanly possible (Baltes, 2006). We are a species constantly exploring and seeing what's next. Undoubtedly, there can be a purpose and a beauty in that. There is also a liability to it. As we push ourselves, we begin to exist beyond human limits. The limit-pushing mindset now applies to more than meaningful endeavors like space travel, physical prowess, or saving the planet. It has seeped into daily functioning, creating an inhabitable set of conditions for most people to maintain with mental wellness.

Advancements in technology also complicate matters. Humanity used to be limited in some capacities by context. The sun would set and no electricity would encourage the end of a work day. I could travel only as far as my legs or horse could carry me, limiting my scope of work and influence. Before the telephone and the cell phone, I was only available to the people in my physical proximity. Fast forward to the present where phones and computers open up the possibility of a twenty-four hour work day. Modern day travel expands the geography of where a person is required to be. At any given moment, there are no limits on the messages received, available information, and expectation for response. It starts to seem reasonable to demand ourselves to do more, be more, and accomplish more.

In my clinical observation, I hear reports of seemingly inexplicable anxiety, a constant on-edge state with calm or rest only happening on vacation or when forced by illness. We may assume that a default way of living that operates beyond human welfare is the norm. It comes with a cost (Walsh, 2011).

Considering Potential

On the other end of the spectrum, there is a suboptimal way of living in which people are increasingly less engaged in their day-to-day living, avoiding not only their limitations but also their full capacity. There is a problem in functioning and in the experience of life when we live in a "discrepancy between potential (or ability) and performance (or achievement)" (Dowdall and Colangelo, 1982).

Not too long ago, I was driving down the highway and I passed a pristine, sleek, expensive sports car. I passed it because it was going at least 10 mph beneath the speed limit. It seemed out of place. A car like that was not meant to dawdle down the road. There can be the same tendency in humans. Leonardo da Vinci explained it like this: "Iron rusts from disuse; stagnant water loses its purity and in cold weather becomes frozen; even so does inaction sap the vigor of the mind. So we must stretch ourselves to the very limits of human possibility" (McCurdy, 1939).

We can shortchange what we are and what we can do. I'm not talking about achievements that are measured on normative scales like grades, income, or influence. Comparison has no place in consideration of potential; it's personal to you and your context. Your personality, abilities, and idiosyncrasies are needed, and the people and places around you may flourish along with your capacity (Ryff, 2018). There's a relationship between not fulfilling what we are capable of and a deterioration of mental health (van Batenburg-Eddes & Jolles, 2013). Indeed, lack of use leads to breakdown.

Considering the Span Between

Span is the optimal quality of life, different for each individual, that is found in tapping into our capacity without betraying our limitations. I came across a distinction in the literature between "lifespan" and "life expectancy". Life expectancy is merely the average number of years we can anticipate in a lifetime; whereas lifespan has a feature of fullness or a "robust" quality within those years (Wachter & Finch, 1997). The proper use of span ensures that the human experience is fully living, with both surprising accomplishment and relieving restraint.

As span involves the conscious use of both potential and limits, there will likely come a time when it may be appropriate to push beyond limits for a cause that matters to you. Clearly identifying values will serve in the decision-making process of how and when to take on the cost of challenging ourselves. There is a time to act, even at a personal cost. Doing so willingly positively correlates with mental well-being (Righetti et al., 2020).

So, we can orient mindlessly to limits, internal resources being leached by the urgency around us. We can orient ourselves indifferently to potential, missing the opportunity to function in the remarkable capacity of our humanity. Or, we can aim for a life that enjoys the fulfillment of sustainably tapping into our capacity, viewing limits as helpful safeguards.

THE SCIENCE OF SPAN

Span is about living fully yet sustainably within limits that honor our humanity. We are more able to extend past limits when it really matters, when it's consistent with our values, if we are regularly living within reasonable limits. There is value to challenging ourselves, to pushing ourselves to do great and necessary things. However, what seems to be the norm is that people have a lifestyle beyond limits in nonmeaningful ways that lead to negative effects on mental health. The constant push will cost the brain-body system, often creating a deficit. Instead of consciously calculating and investing capacity, it's like we have signed up for an ongoing subscription that is automatically taken out even if we aren't benefiting from the service. The result: missing out on the satisfaction of dedicating ourselves where and when it counts or continuing in habits that tax mental health.

Stepping into our humanity and recognizing limits can enhance our mental wellness. At times, there is a disregard for the resource of span, either with a seeming pride at the levels to which we push ourselves or with indifference as if living beneath our potential is inconsequential. On both ends of the spectrum, mental disruption is tied to the neglect of our span. Though span will look distinct for each of us, depending on factors of capacity and factors of limitation, the common thread is that either extreme negatively affects mental health.

Span is the proper functioning of our vessel. Potential is all that we can do. Limits are boundary markers, within which we can flourish and beyond which we deteriorate. Our inclination for mental wellness is found within the kindness of human limits, within our span. **Span provides an optimal structure for human functioning and mental wellness.**

The Negative Effects of Disregarding Limits

What limitations are we talking about? I'm not talking about the limits of ability; if you can't do something, you can't do something. I'm talking about the limits characterized by intended function, the bounds beyond which our condition is compromised. From our cells on up, we are marked by boundaries. In other words, "the human body is a finite organism with structural and functional boundaries" (Marck et al., 2017). Some limits are universal to all humans, while some limits will differ person-to-person. For example, all cars share some limits in operation. They aren't meant for water travel. They don't take flight. However, a smart car and a pickup truck have different capacities. They have some overlap, but both have capabilities the other lacks. The contrasting limits of functioning among people is similar. You will have a different capacity than those around you.

Wherever one's limits are, to mentally go beyond them is damaging to the brain and to daily functioning. Research on the brain indicates that unregulated stress results in impairment of the prefrontal cortex (PFC), the portion of the brain responsible for crucial operations like thought, action, and emotions. The rising levels of norepinephrine and dopamine overwhelm PFC processing (Arnsten & Shanafelt, 2021). The changes are observable in brain circuitry and manifest in deficits in memory, attention, decision-making, and cognition (Liston et al., 2009). Neural connections are compromised and even severed, though they can be restored by reining our functioning back within proper limits.

Overwork and the experience of "time famine," not enough time with too much to do, will cost mental and physical health dearly (Lupu &

Rokka, 2022). Though we may be able to force the body to do something, will ourselves to keep going, we cannot inoculate the brain from the negative effects of such a lifestyle. Indeed, clinical symptoms of a depressive nature may be rooted essentially in working, professionally or domestically, beyond limits. In my clinical observation, some of the most stubborn symptoms of mental illness remain because a lifestyle of overextension will not be negotiated. Often, the idea of scaling back is unthinkable because there are priorities at play that can't be compromised. In protecting that essential priority, there's a hesitancy to evaluate lifestyle. In reality, that which is being protected would be better served by a careful consideration of span.

When we choose to fall back in some areas, we create an increase of targeted effectiveness. I think of a water hose. Without a hose, the water would spill out indiscriminately, some splashing where it's useful but most lost in a puddle. With a hose, the water can be channeled to pour directly where it's intended. Still at other times, a thumb partially covering the opening produces even more constraint, resulting in greater force and accuracing in directing the spray. The water can actually project farther with the restriction than without it. So it seems to be with the human span.

The Positive Effects of Reaching for Potential

Since before the time of Aristotle, those focused on holistic human well-being recognized that there must be a "striving toward an excellence consistent with innate potentialities" (Ryff, 2018). Living beyond human limits distracts from where our true capacity lies. We live, at times, giving our deepest passions and highest values the leftovers of our time and energy, and rarely are there leftovers. As we begin to check ourselves, to acknowledge where as humans our limits exist in our intended functioning, we experience a collecting of our internal capital. The reserves get filled and we can begin to take inventory of our personhood. We can begin drawing connections between what we have available within us and the most important pursuits available to us. As we replenish ourselves, we may see what seemed previously unattainable is actually doable.

Realizing potential is a positive step in living more inline with our values, and yet there is additional benefit in what this does for the human brain and mental wellness. There is research that demonstrates pursuits of engagement and of accomplishment as essential to well-being, much like pleasure or positive relationships. Such endeavors have been seen to improve depressive symptoms for as long as three to six months (Gander, et al., 2016). As the human brain actively invests in projects of purpose, there is a lowering of some cortisol (stress hormone) patterns, as well as positive changes in brain volume resulting in improved functioning (Ryff, 2018).

In hard times, we may view the antidote to stress to be no stress. Unfortunately this may cause patterns of avoidance. Some in the field view "flow" as the optimal counterpart to stress. Flow is described as the "experiences that are most enjoyable in human life while fully engaging in an activity" (Cheron, 2016). Although periods of rest are essential, if they are only momentary pauses between periods of uncontrollable stress, we will not be doing our mental health any favors. The picture painted of optimal span requires action, yet action that is specific, calculated, paced. Such states of flow improve our sense of capability, improve attention networks, and cultivate a supportive sense of self.

In trauma work, we are aware of the ways people numb to escape uncomfortable memories and associations. The numbing can bring relief, and yet numbing after a time produces its own terror and panic, as the self seems to become isolated from engagement in the human experience. The actions we take to numb can be extreme, and the result can be increased damage to the mental state (Burstow, 2003). Even more insidious, we may distract from the actively engaged pursuit of our potential through ongoing, mindless distraction. When distraction, particularly in the form of technology, becomes the default response to stress rather than engagement, there are direct correlations with a disruption in mental health and an increase in anxiety (Panova and Lleras, 2016).

Shortchanging potential may not seem alarming, but it has a dehumanizing effect. Part of harnessing span begins with awareness, interoception, and balance. In daily living, a sensible monitoring, pacing, and applying of our person is paramount.

The Sweet Spot of Span

Living beyond human capacity exhausts our faculties. As humans, there is an innate resilience that's pretty incredible, and it ebbs and flows throughout the lifespan. In a phenomenon called "stress inoculation", research has indicated that greater resilience to stress comes from moderate exposure to adversity throughout adolescence (Feder, et al., 2019). In other words, too much exposure to difficulty leads to more break down; too little exposure to difficulty results in a lack of preparedness for hardship. Our resilience is built by the struggle in life, but by moving through it in doses. Though the sources of our struggles may be beyond our control, the way in which we approach the hardship makes a difference. Again, balance is crucial. Challenge is an asset in fostering resilience, but it can become a liability if approached in an unchecked manner.

The resilience that comes with readily going into challenges or reaching for goals brings with it positive changes in the brain. As the brain goes through the experience of managing a difficult situation or sees that other resources can help us make it through, the prefrontal cortex develops the ability to regulate the stress response and create balance in the neurochemicals at play (Arnsten & Shanafelt, 2021). The mindset in which we engage with these challenges also makes a difference in the experience.

The element of choice alters the experience of times when we may need to push ourselves. There are, of course, aspects of the obstacles in our lives that we do not choose; however, the degree to which we are moving forward of our own volition is important to keep central. The job may be unpleasant, yet one may proactively choose to go because of the income and livelihood it provides for the family. The surgery may be terrifying and the results unknown, yet one may go under willingly for the hopeful chance of healing. The relationship may be in pieces, yet one may stay for love and faithfulness. By focusing on the element of choice, a grounding within span occurs where the limits are respected and conscious engagement is owned. In essence, whether we have a passive or active mindset of control going through hard times will alter how we experience it (Schnell, 2022). In a situation that is unchangeable, the choice to accept and enter in with reasonable pace is transformative.

There may be a temptation to focus on the difficulty we don't control, and ignore the sources of difficulty we do control. In the dynamics of life where we are afforded more free choice, there is an "optimal busyness" of active engagement and proper pacing that produces experiences of elation, energy, well-being (Lupu & Rokka, 2022). To stay in that ideal range requires ongoing adjustments, avoiding the purposelessness of inaction and the burnout of overwork. Potential and limits will oscillate for each person from time to time. Mindful balance in both, a serious regard for limits, and an engaged pursuit of potential can be developed into a lifestyle.

SPAN IN PRACTICE

If mental health is a priority, then perhaps consideration is warranted on whether or not our lifestyle is supportive or taking us beyond where we function optimally. Can we consider if we have adopted a lifestyle that is actually inhumane? Conversely, perhaps comfort, convenience, or discouragement is lulling you into a pace below your potential, leading to dissatisfaction or listlessness. If mental health is a priority, then perhaps you would be invigorated by considering where it would be most meaningful to push yourself in new ways that may be more natural to you than you realize. Can we consider if we have assumed a lifestyle that is accidentally subhuman?

Living in a way that draws from our span rather than spoiling it can be difficult. The following practices focus on awareness and proper use of both our potential and our limits, ushering us into a use of span that cultivates mental wellness. **We practice span with a clarifying balance of recognized limits and purposeful potential.**

Meditation Practice – A Meditation on Noticing Span

The following meditation focuses on limits and potential, while also noticing the discomfort that can come with changing either. It may be a new experience to find calm in acknowledging limits or in pushing potential. Using visualization and options for gentle movement, allow your mind to reapproach your consideration of span. Go to kristaagler.com/book/keepinmind to listen to the provided audio or follow the accompanying prompts for a guided meditation on mindful observation of span.

Reflection Practice – Examining Limitation and Potential

The goal is not restriction for its own sake; the aim is liberation to do what matters most. By closing off nonmeaningful channels of output, we can grow the capacity of what we can do. Honestly examining and responding to limits may reframe our prospects. Respond to the prompts in Table 5.1 to practically examine your limits and your potential. Honesty and nonjudgment are good starting points for accurately assessing limits.

Conscious Practice – Harnessing Span: A Time Study

A time study is a practice to gain insight into where our capacity is actually going. The practical impact of this practice is profound. A time study tracks where time is going and evaluates the alignment of that time spent with a value-based objective. Life becomes disjointed when we're going through motions that aren't producing the good we want. We each have the same twenty-four hour period each day, and a look at how we're spending that universal capital helps reorient us toward a more fulfilling lifestyle.

In tracking time, we can see the ways in which our efforts are going toward what is necessary: work to provide for the self and others, stewarding our bodies and homes, and so forth. We can also see the optional uses of

Table 5.1 *Examining Limitation and Potential*

Examining Limitations: *In considering the following prompts, consider all areas of life: time, work, energy, finances, social relationships, hobbies, personality, homelife, schedule, physical ability, etc.*	
Prompt	**Response**
What in my life seems unsustainable?	
Where would I experience relief if I were given permission to stop, opt out, or pause?	
What does it seem others can do that I just can't?	
At what times am I most exhausted or likely to get sick?	
Examining Potential: In considering the following prompts, brainstorm answers with no holds barred; anything and everything is on the table.	
Prompt	**Response**
What value is most important to me, and what would I do if it could be my top priority? Consider multiple values as well.	
What is the highest hope you have of what could characterize your life, and what could you do that is consistent with that characterization?	
How could you reapproach regular, necessary tasks in daily life if you had more energy and time? How would those tasks improve?	
What activities or endeavors come to your mind often that would be beneficial for you, for others, and for the world around you?	

time and evaluate how that use of time functions in our life, how it makes us feel, and what it is actually accomplishing. We can learn a lot from a time study.

The task before you now is to complete a time study. Below is a time sheet. Note: a.m. and p.m. are not marked so that the time sheet can be used by those on night shift as well as day shift workers. Track how your time is spent, being as specific as you can. So, instead of filling in eight hours with "work," note time spent on "work emails", "optional meeting," "social interactions with coworkers," and so forth. If keeping track as you go is too cumbersome, revisit your time sheet every two or three hours, making notes retroactively.

At the end of the week, read it over and evaluate: What in the week absolutely has to happen? And what is optional? What is consistent with your values? Where are you spending time because it's important to others? If you could take one optional thing away, what would it be? What

Table 5.2 *Harnessing Span: A Time Study*

	Sunday	*Monday*	*Tuesday*	*Wednesday*	*Thursday*	*Friday*	*Saturday*
12:00							
1:00							
2:00							
3:00							
4:00							
5:00							
6:00							
7:00							
8:00							
9:00							
10:00							
11:00							
12:00							
1:00							
2:00							
3:00							
4:00							
5:00							
6:00							
7:00							
8:00							
9:00							
10:00							
11:00							

necessary or beneficial activities are lacking time in your week? What patterns do you notice? If you could change one thing, what would you change? What's the worst part of the week? What's the best part? Note which activities drain your energy and which replenish it. Use these questions to gain awareness.

Finally, make changes in accordance with your values, prioritizing the essential and the beneficial. What will you stop? What will you reduce? What needs to be adjusted? What could be added? There will likely be a shift in mental wellness just by acknowledging limits and reapplying capacity.

Lifestyle Practice – Practicing "No" and a Better "Yes"

Think of span in terms of percentages. You can't give something 110%. By definition, you only have 100% to give, in total. You can't give 100% to your marriage or to your job or to your art or to your healing. You have

Table 5.3 *Practicing "No" and a Better "Yes"*

Identify activities receiving too high a percentage of your capacity.	**Identify the specific "no" that would reclaim part of the percentage.**	**Identify the specific "yes" that is possible with the newly acquired percentage.**
Example: Staying late at work to try to get ahead	Example: "I will not stay past my contracted time unless by specific, rare exception."	Example: "I will use the extra time to commute to work by bike, which is a passion and value."

to divide it among each one. You are spending percentages with each choice of where you exert time, energy, and self. Mental disruption can come from using percentages where they don't belong, even if they are seemingly good pursuits. Saying no reclaims some of your percentage and is like money in your pocket. Better actually.

Saying no is essential. It is the preamble to your better "yes." Everything you say no to creates blank space for you to invest your percentages more effectively. Refer to Table 5.3 and consider: What activities are unintentionally taking too much of your percentages? Consider if maybe they shouldn't be taking any at all. Identify these activities. Then, identify the specific "no" and the specific "yes" that would redistribute those percentages. You can say yes to placing your time, energy, and resources in better alignment with your values. You have more control than you may realize, and your absent "yes" may be as problematic to your mental wellness as your absent "no."

IN SUMMARY

You have reasons, conscious or subconscious, for why you have allowed your time, energy, and self to be divvied out the way it is now. It will likely be uncomfortable to go against it, to make a change in how you steward the resource of your span. There's the discomfort of the way things are, or there's the discomfort of change. Mental wellness flourishes when limits are respected and potential is activated. Coming back into your limits in order to connect with your potential is an ongoing, intentional practice. You will be required to use choice and pursue balance to steward your span throughout life. Span invites us to come back, again and again, into what we are: a dynamic, limited yet untapped human being.

REFERENCES

Arnsten, A. F., & Shanafelt, T. (2021). Physician distress and burnout: The neurobiological perspective. *Mayo Clinic Proceedings, 96*(3), 763–769.

Baltes, P. B. (2006). Facing our limits: human dignity in the very old. *Daedalus, 135*(1), 32–39.

Burstow, B. (2003). Toward a radical understanding of trauma and trauma work. *Violence Against Women, 9*(11), 1293–1317.

Cheron, G. (2016). How to measure the psychological "flow"? A neuroscience perspective. *Frontiers in Psychology, 7*, 1823.

Dowdall, C. B., & Colangelo, N. (1982). Underachieving gifted students: review and implications. *Gifted Child Quarterly, 26*(4), 179–84.

Feder, A., Fred-Torres, S., Southwick, S. M., & Charney, D. S. (2019). The biology of human resilience: Opportunities for enhancing resilience across the life span. *Biological Psychiatry, 86*(6), 443–453.

Gander, F., Proyer, R. T., & Ruch, W. (2016). Positive psychology interventions addressing pleasure, engagement, meaning, positive relationships, and accomplishment increase well-being and ameliorate depressive symptoms: A randomized, placebo-controlled online study. *Frontiers in Psychology, 7,* 686.

Liston, C., McEwen, B. S., & Casey, B. J. (2009). Psychosocial stress reversibly disrupts prefrontal processing and attentional control. *Proceedings of the National Academy of Sciences, 106*(3), 912–917.

Lupu, I., & Rokka, J. (2022). "Feeling in control": Optimal busyness and the temporality of organizational controls. *Organization Science, 33*(4), 1396–1422.

Marck, A., Antero, J., Berthelot, G., Saulière, G., Jancovici, J.-M., Masson-Delmotte, V., Boeuf, G., Spedding, M., Le Bourg, É., & Toussaint, J.-F. (2017). Are we reaching the limits of homo sapiens? *Frontiers in Physiology, 8,* 812–812.

McCurdy, E. (Ed.). (1939). *The notebooks of Leonardo da Vinci.* George Braziller.

Panova, T., & Lleras, A. (2016). Avoidance or boredom: Negative mental health outcomes associated with use of Information and Communication Technologies depend on users' motivations. *Computers in Human Behavior, 58,* 249–258.

Righetti, F., Sakaluk, J. K., Faure, R., & Impett, E. A. (2020). The link between sacrifice and relational and personal well-being: A meta-analysis. *Psychological Bulletin, 146*(10), 900.

Ryff, C. D. (2018). Well-being with soul: Science in pursuit of human potential. *Perspectives on psychological science: A Journal of the Association for Psychological Science, 13*(2), 242–248.

Schnell, T. (2022). Suffering as meaningful choice. An existential approach. *Ta vare. En bok om diakoni, sjelesorg og eksistensiell helse,* 3–14.

van Batenburg-Eddes, T., & Jolles, J. (2013). How does emotional wellbeing relate to underachievement in a general population sample of young adolescents: A neurocognitive perspective. *Frontiers in Psychology, 4.*

Wachter, K. W., & Finch, C. E. (Eds.). (1997). *Between Zeus and the salmon: The biodemography of longevity* (1st ed.). National Academy Press.

Walsh, R. (2011). Lifestyle and mental health. *American Psychologist, 66*(7), 579.

PART II

EXTERNAL RESOURCES

Chapter 6

Body: A Resource of Movement Messaging

At thirty-two years old, Heath was not concerned about his mental health. He was concerned about the rising cost of housing, and he was concerned about taking good care of his dog. He worried about politics, and he had recently begun worrying about his physical health. Mental health had never been a problem for him. He worked remotely, lived an adventurously active lifestyle, and kept to himself for the most part.

He grew up in a small town – everyone knew everyone. When he was young, from the age of eight until eleven, he was physically and sexually mistreated by a prominent man within their small community. Heath never told a soul. He would later say that he accepted it as part of his history, and he closed it away, under lock and key. He would wonder from time to time if those years of abuse were partly to blame for his tendency to isolate, the difficulty he had keeping a girlfriend, or close friends for that matter. Still, he had grown accustomed to it and had "made peace."

Shortly after his thirtieth birthday, he began to get sick. It started with his digestion in the form of debilitating pain. He remained active but noticed he was losing the wrong kind of weight along with his strength. He began to develop patches of itchy skin, which was maddening, and a pain in his jaw that he often felt at night began to ache twenty-four hours a day. He went to doctors, underwent extensive testing, addressed potential allergies, and tried a variety of supplements and medications until finally the doctors concluded it was "psychosomatic."

Heath went to therapy, skeptical and sheepish. To think his physical symptoms were "all in his head" felt almost insulting, and he recoiled from the idea of talking about himself or his feelings. Following the doctors' consensus that there was a psychological component to his physical symptoms, the therapist explained to Heath the ways they could be addressed.

DOI: 10.4324/9781003521945-9

When asked about a trauma history, he declined to share what happened when he was a boy. He was still convinced it had nothing to do with what his body was experiencing. The therapist directed him to responsive practices to the physical symptoms.

Determined to show the doctors they were wrong, he agreed to try a specific therapy, Eye Movement Desensitization and Reprocessing (EMDR), that focused on the physical symptom of his jaw pain. In short order, he discovered the jaw pain was rooted in harmful experiences he had during the years of sustained abuse. To his credit, he continued with the EMDR sessions until he had thoroughly addressed those painful memories and the stubborn ache that stretched from chin to ears all but vanished. The ongoing responsive practices were showing promise as his itchy skin and stomach problems were slowly but steadily improving. Heath would summarize it in this way: "I guess my body wasn't able to hold in what I thought my heart and mind should." Well said.

THE NATURE OF THE BODY

As a mental health therapist, the implications of body-based healing of the brain always held deep fascination for me. I began incorporating small, holistic, body-based suggestions for clients who were interested and was pleased with the results. Eventually, I received training in EMDR therapy, a trauma therapy using movement or bilateral (intermittent on both sides of the body) stimulation with a shockingly positive outcome.

I am suspicious of silver bullets or cure-alls. Largely, mental health treatment is hard work for clients – no shortchanging that. However, after years of the slow-but-steady pace of counseling, the leaps forward that came for my clients with EMDR was exhilarating. Though these therapies and interventions are valuable and certainly worth pursuing, what excites me most is that the key resource in these changes is not the therapy itself but something that rests with the client: their own body.

For Heath, his nervous system was communicating through his skin and digestion. That's not random or rare. The brain and the body are communicating with each other and through each other at all times (Shapiro, 2012). We splice them apart to understand them better, but they don't stop influencing each other. "The separation of mind and body, however, is a theoretical construct - well represented in our daily language and thought patterns, but quite unsubstantiated in fact" (Bentzen et al., 2004). The exchange between brain and body, body and brain is more like the constant contact of two-seeming-as-one dancing the tango than staccato turn taking of walkie-talkies. The connection is well established and serves a profound purpose for mental wellness. **The body is a constant resource,**

available to provide firsthand insight, direct feedback, and real time course correction.

Brain Manifested in Body

As we see the intertwined nature of brain and body, mental health is undeniably demonstrated in the body. For example, there is an established bidirectional feedback loop signaling between nerves of the nervous system and skin cells through neuropeptides (Choi & Di Nardo, 2018). The dynamic between the skin and the nervous system is intricately woven together. Itching can be one manifestation of the interplay between the two (Caccavale et al., 2016). Similarly, interactive messaging is seen between the stomach and the mind, in communication occurring between stress responses and the balance in the microbiome of the gut (Holzer et al., 2017). More generally, symptoms of depression are at times experienced and described as physical heaviness, muscle fatigue, and loss of appetite, while symptoms of anxiety are noted in heart rate, muscle tension, or difficulty breathing. These are just a few of the more common ways our bodies display the state of the mind.

Our bodies will continue to experience some symptoms of a traumatic event long after it has ended (Shapiro, 2012). Some of these symptoms are indirectly caused, an ongoing expression of the toll the event took on the body's holistic system. Other symptoms are directly linked, a physical reexperiencing of the event. There is a time-lapse associated with unresolved trauma so the brain and body cannot completely differentiate between the past and the present. The body may actually be in one place but physiologically responding to another place and time.

The body is not just the landscape where these symptoms pop-up, as is sometimes too simply assumed. It is also a very powerful platform through which we move beyond the current mental state, whether or not that state is caused by trauma. The body is able to both hold information and influence state. It is constant in its present and active role in containing and connecting our mind with our experience of life.

Consideration of Weakness and Limits

And yet, our bodies are often broken, sick, or strained. For many, perhaps for most, there are real, pervasive, and even debilitating limitations to the body. It's true that some will have seemingly more available to them from the resource of the body than others. A couple considerations to that point: One, you may shift to a perspective of drawing from what is available rather than viewing what is not available. A small investment brings back dividends. A subtle strength is still strength. Draw from and use what you can. It may do more than you think. Two, many have found that focusing for a time on the place of pain, limitation, or disability is a source of added strength, though that may not be available or desirable to everyone. It is worth considering, and I invite you to do so.

By considering the whole body – strengths and weaknesses – as a resource for mental wellness, we can transmute what seemed a liability or nonfactor into a catalyst for available, sustainable change.

THE SCIENCE OF THE BODY

Our physical bodies are the infrastructure through which we can exercise control of a meaningful portion of even involuntary systems. Consider any fully functioning community: there are communication channels, walkways and/or roadways, routes by which food is transported, and the like. All of this is possible by infrastructure. The physical body, even with limitations, hosts commonplace means by which we have sway over many organs and systems. **The body provides highly intuitive, interactive messaging that can be directed for improved mental wellness**.

Interoception, Once Again

Our previous discussion of interoception in the chapter on existence focused on the role it plays in the prefrontal cortex in establishing our sense of self. Part of what makes the body such a ready and powerful resource is the amount of voluntary control we have over it. Interoception is one route through which we can maximize use of the governable body (Todd & Aspell, 2022). In other words, the ways in which you can control your specific body are ways in which you can positively support mental health. Where we lack functioning of our body, we can allow others to help us incorporate these movements. Our focus will be on the ways interoception can be tangibly engaged. In all of it, a growing awareness of and attention to the body's experience in connection to mental health is key.

"Interoception refers to the process by which the nervous system senses, interprets, and integrates signals originating from within the body, providing a moment-by-moment mapping of the body's internal landscape across conscious and unconscious levels" (Khalsa et al., 2018). Just as we have the well-known exteroceptive senses to take in information from what is around us, we have the ability to take in information from what is within us (Schmitt & Schoen, 2022). Although most occurs unconsciously, the conscious portions are of great value in the work of improving mental wellness. We can extract accessible parts of interoception through "attentional focus" (Khalsa et al., 2018), and we do so by directing attention to the resource of the body in particular ways that can be practiced readily.

Disruptions of interoception are linked to a variety of mental health problems, such as mood and anxiety disorders (Khalsa et al., 2018). Think about it. A generalized disruption to our exteroceptive senses could lead to disorientation. If you are a person who relies on glasses to see and finds them missing, you know what I'm talking about. It follows that a disconnection to the messaging available within could also lead to disordering.

Interoception is the process of sensing and feeling with attentional focus in order to understand what's going on in and around us through our bodies. It is from interoception that we select responses (Schmitt & Shoen, 2022). I take off my jacket when I register my body is heating up. I realize it's time for lunch because my mind translates signals from my body that I'm hungry. I get a tingly sensation on the back of my neck as I enter a situation that is typically overwhelming to me, so I take a deep breath. All interoception at work. These examples are the low-hanging fruit. There are more nuanced multitudes of ways our bodies are communicating with us constantly.

Interoception is the awareness that precedes regulation. Although it can function imperceptibly, we can also nurture awareness of and connection to our bodies to gain a wealth of information. Temperature, skin sensations, balance, hunger, muscle tension, and others are all informants from within our bodies about the present moment.

Specific to mental health, interoception can provide us with information about mood regulation, awareness of perceived or actual threat, sensitivity to stress or difficulty, readiness for challenge, motivation, growing heat in response to injustice, and passages of grief, just to name a few. We pick up these indicators from our bodies. In understanding our body as a resource, I want us to see it as a messenger that is ready to serve the mind by responding to information gathered through interoception.

Movement for Mental Health

Muscles and the movement of the body can build into our mental wellness. It is well established that physical activity is good for our mental health. The goal of "movement" instead of "fitness" or "working out" may be beneficial for mental health as it may be more accessible. For mental-wellness purposes, a "lifestyle" of movement outranks a specific fitness regimen or protocol (Parker et al., 2008). On the one hand, moving more consistently is beneficial, while on the other hand, there are intentional movements that directly serve mental wellness.

The term "movement" centralizes a function that can be carried out throughout all of life and serves to integrate the body into nonphysical arenas. Here, the focus on movement is not fitness, but specific movements for specific mental health benefits.

Body-to-Brain Messaging

The body not only receives messages from the brain but also sends messages to it. The manipulation of our muscles, particularly through movement and muscle control, is a powerful messenger. There is increasing awareness of how "emotions and cognitions are associated with muscular states, including facial expressions, body postures, and movements" (Hackford et al., 2019).

The role of movement is immediate and crucial in the work of regulation. The way we hold and carry our bodies is an indicator of brain state. It's a manifestation of a message received by the brain. High shoulders or a bouncing leg can indicate anxiety. Drooping shoulders and slow movement can suggest depressive symptoms. However, the messaging goes both ways. Relaxing muscles and releasing shoulders can send a message to the brain that we are allowed to be calm. Straightening the posture can similarly participate in the interoceptive brain-body communication loop and send a message to the brain to shift the mood in a positive direction (Nair et al., 2015). Even the manner in which we walk, a more jaunty stride or a heavy lumber, directly impacts the connections happening in the brain, how we perceive things, and so then how we feel and behave (Hackford et al., 2019).

Movements are an intentional invitation from the body to the brain to consider options, to try a new or additional way of being. So it could go like this: The brain takes in data and decides the situation, such as an outstanding bill coming in the mail, is a threat. It sends thought messages and it also sends physical messages like shortening the breath slightly or tension in the neck. The messages say to and through the body, "Be on alert. This is a threat." The body in that state receives and has potential to reinforce that message of threat. However, perhaps after assessing the situation, it is decided that the situation can be handled. Intentional muscle movements can then be initiated, regulating the body and sending the message to the brain to still the alarm.

It may be surprising to learn that specific muscle groups in the body are closely connected to mental health processes. For example, the pelvic floor is involved in processing emotions, and its activation correlates with stress states (Kasper-Jędrzejewska, 2023). By learning to regulate some of the tension in the pelvic floor, we can support processing of emotions and encourage regulation. Similarly, studies reveal correlations between higher experiences of stress and muscle tension in the jaw (Zieliński et al., 2021). Furthermore, muscles throughout the body are communicating with the brain regarding state of being. By directly manipulating the muscles to a neutral state, in practices such as progressive muscle relaxation, effects are reported to be as positive and almost as swift as fast-acting benzodiazepine psychotropics (Holland et al., 1991). Each of these communication loops have direct access to the brain and are within each individual's influence. Professional intervention is not required to use the body to powerfully alter brain states. Body-to-brain messaging can become a vital part of mental wellness for all.

Bilateral Movement and Crossing the Midline

Bilateral stimulation comes through either movements or sensations that occur intermittently on one side of the body than the other. It is a key component of EMDR, a highly effective and researched therapy built for trauma recovery, yet useful in the wide scope of mental health treatment. Most practitioners of EMDR view bilateral stimulation as the distinctive function of the therapy, engaging a specific part of the brain and thus aiding in the healing process. Additionally, there are those who have done research demonstrating that there is also a healing effect with EMDR as it divides attention from the troubling aspects of a memory or experience through movement, thus relieving suffering (van den Hout & Engelhard, 2012).

We each have a mental scaffolding by which we orient inwardly and outwardly. It's how we make sense of the world. For consistently improving mental wellness, we want that framework to be adaptive. Among other things, this framework is shaped by our past experiences, and those experiences along with their messages are held by memory both conscious and unconscious (Shapiro, 2012). Memories are central in mental health, as they are a key component of all information processing (Hasson et al., 2015).

One way we improve mental wellness is to improve processing of past experiences, whether or not it is considered "trauma," and to improve our relationship to those experiences. In the brain, the corpus callosum, which serves as a kind of bridge between brain hemispheres, is part of that processing (Shapiro, 2012), and it's the part of the brain activated by bilateral stimulation.

The corpus callosum is like a canal, easing access between two oceans, except instead of bodies of water it connects the right and left hemisphere of the brain (Goldstein, et al., 2023). It's a seemingly small channel connecting two larger bodies yet serving a vital purpose between the two. For this reason, I like to refer to the corpus callosum as the brain canal. The brain, including the corpus callosum, is plastic, meaning it retains the ability to change. Use it or lose it, the saying goes. The corpus callosum, the canal, demonstrates the ability for structural change throughout the lifespan due in part to redirection and something called "pruning" (Luders et al., 2010), which is the clearing out of neural connections that go unused. Bilateral stimulation, or activation of each side of the body intermittently, utilizes the "brain canal," keeping it in use and increasing its availability for refining experiences, memories, and other essential connections. That means it's not only a powerful aspect of the notable, effective EMDR therapy but it's also accessible mental health in day-to-day living.

Connecting both hemispheres of the brain isn't just for the isolated benefit of the "canal." It goes beyond the confines of the brain in our skull and affects the central nervous system (CNS). Turns out our entire body plays host to points where we are "cross wired," nerves running perpendicular from the direction from which they came. You may be familiar with the way the brain hemispheres correlate with the opposite side of the body, such as when a stroke occurring on the right hemisphere of the brain impacts use of the left arm. These crossings happen throughout the CNS, impacting many aspects of our bodies such as sensory processing and motor use (Vulliemoz et al., 2005). Bilateral movement and crossing the midline supports not only the corpus callosum, but also the entire nervous system. Francine Shapiro, the originator of EMDR, wrote a book for people to utilize some of the skills used formally in therapy in everyday life. She describes an approach of crossing the arms and alternatively tapping opposite shoulders, in a movement she calls "the butterfly hug" (Shapiro, 2012). It is a simple movement, but necessarily supplemental for our brains that are deprived of such physical input.

Increasingly, the modern lifestyle may hinder a healthy, regular use of natural cross-body movement. Over generations the functioning of our daily movement has shifted dramatically (Kahn et al., 2020), not only in amount but also in form. Prior to much of modernization, there was ample opportunity and need for nuanced movement including cross-body movement: rowing a boat, washing clothes by hand, building and farming without modern tools, horseback riding, and the like all naturally require crossing the midline or bilateral stimulation. Now, our movements are often much more parallel: hands on left and right of the keyboard, hands ten-and-two on the steering wheel, and general sedentary posturing decreases the natural opportunities for keeping the corpus callosum maintained and in good use. Intentionality in cross lateral movement and stimulation meets a basic, simple need.

By crossing the midline in movement, we are not only activating the brain, we are also supporting points along our CNS to be in good working order. That movement initiates a brain-and-body activation of mindful, here-and-now existence, surpassing the sentiment or emotion of "being mindful," and making it a physiological reality. Reminders of the problematic past can pull us out of the relevance of what is happening now, especially as the effects of some memories or some learned patterns can be exceptionally strong. By thinking about various "past-points" making up our framework while simultaneously engaging in cross lateral movement, we can "tax" our working memory of those "past-points," lessening the intensity and rerouting that energy to the less problematic present (van den Hout & Engelhard, 2012). Simple movements that provide bilateral stimulation while also crossing the midline, when done mindfully, remedy both past stuck points as well as immediate disturbances.

BODY IN PRACTICE

For mental wellness, our body is part of a mutual exchange with the brain and can be brought into alignment with our values and an upward mental health trajectory. **We practice with the body by building a lifestyle of body awareness and micromovements that respond adaptively to and for mental health**. These can be gentle shifts rather than hardcore goals. To attune to the messages of interoception and respond with sustainable movement is to champion for yourself a truly holistic mental health.

A crucial note before we continue: these movement practices, in some form, are available to everyone. Even if someone cannot complete these movements themselves, bilateral stimulation or cross-lateral movement can be offered by another. Parents of children, caregivers, partners, and friends can all assist in administering these movements for someone else. Some options for modifications of the following practices are offered; however, where it's not possible to extensively provide such options for each nuanced, unique body, I hope the options offered provide some brainstorming to adjust them for how it may work for you. Going outside of the box may make the practices even more effective.

Meditation Practice – A Guided Meditation on Interoception and Attentional Focus

Directing attention to the external and interoceptive cues coming from the body increases the synchronization between brain and body. Increasing the skill of understanding what's going on in your body and what messages it is relaying, can be pivotal to a lifestyle of mental wellness. Go to kristaagler.com/book/keepinmind to listen to the provided audio or follow the accompanying prompts for a guided meditation on interoception and attentional focus.

Reflection Practice – Connecting Your Body and Your Mental Health

Our bodies, whether healthy or not and broken or not, are the mediums through which we experience life. Consider, how does your unique body, as it is today, shape and inform your experience? What nuances of your physical body are individual to you? Though it may be difficult, I invite you to consider and appreciate the painful or limiting aspects of your physical body. The whole body, the weak parts and the strong, are an asset for your mental wellness.

It's been said that "our bodies are apt to be our autobiographies" (Burgess, 1942). What does the experience of your body-and-brain connection indicate about your past, your present, and your future? The inseparable relationship between brain and body exists whether we welcome it or not. By applying the previously used double-storied practices specifically to the body, use Table 6.1 to improve the quality of awareness of the brain-body connection.

Conscious Practice – Practice Crossing Midline and Bilateral Stimulation

The brain benefits from simple movements that cross the midline while providing bilateral stimulation. With my clients, I typically refer to the process as "cross-shoulder tapping." An intuitive movement, its use isn't primarily for therapy, but for day-to-day living. The benefits of activating the "brain canal" are immediately accessible and intrinsic to the human system.

Prepare by setting apart some time, could be as little as five minutes, but could stretch to fifteen. A timer may be helpful. Turn down other sounds and minimize distractions. Quiet and alone is best for this practice.

Step 1 – Cross and Tap

Cross your arms, placing one hand on each shoulder. Tap one shoulder and then the other, continuing at a slow to moderate pace. The general rule: The slower the tapping, the more calming; the more rapid the tapping,

Table 6.1 Connecting Your Body and Your Mental Health

<table>
<tr><th>Past Prompt</th><th>Response</th></tr>
<tr><td>Identify three weaknesses or limits of your physical body.</td><td></td></tr>
<tr><td>Identify five strengths or comforts of your physical body.</td><td></td></tr>
<tr><td colspan="2">Direction: Fill in the blanks below, pairing strengths with weaknesses.</td></tr>
<tr><td colspan="2">Example:
My body has been characterized both by pain and endurance, by insecurity

and walking my dog, and by violation and creative movement.</td></tr>
<tr><td colspan="2">Your response:
My body has been characterized by ______________ and ______________, ______________ and ______________, ______________ and ______________
______.</td></tr>
<tr><td>Present Prompt</td><td>Response</td></tr>
<tr><td>Identify a current life obstacle or struggle.</td><td></td></tr>
<tr><td>Identify a mental health benefit that would come with any improvement.</td><td></td></tr>
<tr><td>Identify a current bodily ability, asset, or support at your disposal.</td><td></td></tr>
<tr><td colspan="2">Direction: Use the above responses to fill in the blanks to form neural connections to see the body as an active support to mental health.</td></tr>
<tr><td colspan="2">Example:
Even though my work is overwhelming, I could experience some peace and relief by walking at the end of each day.</td></tr>
<tr><td colspan="2">Your response:
Even though ______________________, I could experience ______________
_____

by______________________.</td></tr>
</table>

the more activating. Tap for a brief period of time: Ten taps on both sides, or fifteen seconds, or until a pause is desired. That is one set.

Step 2 – Pause and Notice

Keeping your hands on your shoulders, cease tapping for some time. Notice. Notice thoughts, body sensations, anything else that comes to your attention. In this practice, the focus should not be on doing it "right or wrong"; the goal is to honestly notice all that comes up in your brain-body experience. The movement practice and attentional focus is of benefit regardless of how it "feels."

Step 3 – Repeat and Observe

When you feel ready, do another set of tapping. Repeat steps 1 and 2 until your five-to-fifteen minutes is up. Take a few minutes to observe any final thoughts, emotions, body sensations. Observe any changes in your demeanor, mindset, or mood. Transition mindfully from the practice back to the normal events of the day.

Modification: If this movement is unavailable or uncomfortable for you, you can create the movement with your eyes. Find a fixed point at eye level and between 10 and 30 feet away. From that point, scan your eyes as far as is comfortable to the right, and then the same to the left before returning to the fixed point. Continue in fluid scans back-and-forth, following the steps above.

Perhaps use of your eyes is not available or advisable for you, but perhaps you have a partner, friend, or caregiver who would support you in this practice. They can provide the "cross tapping" either on your shoulders or knees while you're seated. Have them use the above description to guide you through the bilateral stimulation.

Lifestyle Practice – Body-to-Brain Messaging: Movements for Calming or Activating

Body-to-brain muscle techniques can be readily used as we go through daily life. By using voluntary control of muscles, movement, posture, and so forth, there is an innate ability to engage mental health with the body.

Relax the core muscles – According to Eric Gentry, PhD, by relaxing the muscles of the core, the nervous system immediately shifts from the alarm of the sympathetic state to the calm of the parasympathetic (Gentry, 2022). By doing this, we are able to regain neocortical functioning. In other words, the part of your brain that best serves day-to-day activity is back in the driver's seat. Before going further, it should be acknowledged that use of these core muscles could be triggering to some. If so, take your time warming to the idea, go slow, and yet move steadily toward reclaiming these muscles from past experience and recover their profound role in your mental and holistic health. Relaxation of the core, due to its central location and connection to the entire system's nerves, muscles, and so on is one of the most efficient body-to-brain practices.

To relax the core, find a place to sit on a soft surface. With your hands, find the front of your hip bones and make mental note of that point, like a somatic imprint. Then, sit on your hands, noticing the contact between them and your sitz bones, or the part of your pelvic bone in most direct contact with the sitting surface. Once again, make a mental note of that point. Now, imagine connecting those four points to form a kind of boundary. Everything within that boundary we are going to consider the core. Direct attention to releasing the muscles within that boundary. You will likely notice a tendency for the muscles within that quadrant to immediately contract as soon as attention is not directed at relaxation. That is okay. For a minute, cycle through releasing the muscles repeatedly. By directing attention to even slight loosening of strategic muscles, you keep the best of your brain engaged, encourage the nervous system to calm and regulate the entire system.

Relax the jaw – With a simple movement of the tongue, the jaw can be disengaged. It not only releases tension that could be sending a message to the brain that increases cortisol or an alarm state, it also gives a neutral facial expression. The neutrality sends a message to your brain that whatever is before you may not be "good" or "bad." It gives room for slowing down and gathering more data.

To relax your jaw, close your mouth softly. Touch your tongue to the back of your front-upper teeth. From there, use the tongue to trace along the top of the mouth, following the roof of the mouth back until you reach the soft beginning of the throat. That movement of the tongue disengages the jaw, releasing tension and sending messages of calm, slowing, even problem-solving, and composure.

Straight posture while sitting – A slight shift in posture sends energizing and activating messages to the brain. Find a place to sit, mindfully giving attention to how you're feeling now: energy levels, muscle fatigue, mood, and so forth. Then, mindfully place your feet flat on the floor, giving notice to all the contact between your feet and the ground. Line up your knees, square hips, and then on an inhale, straighten your spine not to be rigid, but to extend to its full, natural height. Allow the top of your head to pull up toward the ceiling. On an exhale, drop the shoulders and soften muscle tension while maintaining the posture. See below for modification.

Walking with a lifted chest – Particularly in response to stressors, or events that raise cortisol levels, walking with a lifted chest rather than slumped shoulders has been seen to demonstrate improvements to psychological and physiological states (Hackford et al., 2019). It is a practice that only requires a handful of steps. The focus here is form, not distance, which provides a message to the brain of readiness and fortitude.

Draw from the previous practice and for a straightened posture. As you prepare to take a few steps, on an inhale, allow your shoulders to pull back and your chest to lift just slightly. It should not be exaggerated or feel inauthentic. It is a slight micromovement. The slight adjustment to your spine, shoulders, and chest will alter your stride in a way that is hardly observable, yet with internal and interoceptive effect.

Modification: If sitting or walking postures are not available to you, focus on one part of the body that is available to you. Give all attention to that part of the body taking on a posture of being lifted. Perhaps lifting the chin and feeling the strength and engagement in the connecting jaw and neck. Perhaps the muscles around the elbows, linking with the forearms or biceps, can be activated and so send the same message to the brain. Whatever is available to you, explore micromovements in that region of the body, noticing what may bring that desired increase of energy and confidence, even if just marginally.

IN SUMMARY

The body, with its form and function, is a powerful complement to the mind in pursuing mental health. By cultivating a view of the body as favorable and essential in brain health, we can begin to see our physical vessel as an asset, even with weaknesses and injuries. At its most basic level, the body holds the ability to participate in mental wellness. With small, simple movements and postures, we hold the ability to take part in the ongoing conversation already happening between the brain and the body, for the better.

REFERENCES

Bentzen, M., Jarlnaes, E., & Levine, P. (2004) The Body Self in Psychotherapy: A psychomotoric approach to developmental psychology. In I. Macnaughton (Ed.), *Body, breath, & consciousness: A somatics anthology: a collection of articles on family systems, self-psychology, the bodynamics model of somatic developmental psychology, shock trauma and breathwork* (pp. 51–70). North Atlantic Books.

Burgess, G. (1942). *Look eleven years younger.* World Pub.

Caccavale, S., Bove, D., Bove, R. M., & LA Montagna, M. (2016). Skin and brain: Itch and psychiatric disorders. *Giornale italiano di dermatologia e venereologia: Organo ufficiale, Societa italiana di dermatologia e sifilografia, 151*(5), 525–529.

Choi, J. E., & Di Nardo, A. (2018). Skin neurogenic inflammation. *Seminars in Immunopathology, 40*(3), 249–259.

Gentry, E. (2022). *Forward-Facing Trauma Therapy: Healing the moral wound.* Outskirts Press.

Goldstein, A., Covington, B. P., Mahabadi, N., Mesfin, F. B. (2023) Neuroanatomy, Corpus Callosum. StatPearls Publishing.

Hackford, J., Mackey, A., & Broadbent, E. (2019). The effects of walking posture on affective and physiological states during stress. *Journal of Behavior Therapy and Experimental Psychiatry, 62,* 80–87.

Hasson, U., Chen, J., & Honey, C. J. (2015). Hierarchical process memory: memory as an integral component of information processing. *Trends in Cognitive Sciences, 19*(6), 304–313.

Holland, J. C., Morrow, G. R., Schmale, A., Derogatis, L., Stefanek, M., Berenson, S., & Feldstein, M. (1991). A randomized clinical trial of alprazolam versus progressive muscle relaxation in cancer patients with anxiety and depressive symptoms. *Journal of Clinical Oncology, 9*(6), 1004–1011.

Holzer, P., Farzi, A., Hassan, A. M., Zenz, G., Jačan, A., & Reichmann, F. (2017). Visceral inflammation and immune activation stress the brain. *Frontiers in Immunology, 8,* 1613.

Kahn, S., Ehrlich, P., Feldman, M., Sapolsky, R., & Wong, S. (2020). The jaw epidemic: Recognition, origins, cures, and prevention. *Bioscience, 70*(9), 759–771.

Kasper-Jędrzejewska, M. (2023, March 14). Consequences of high tension in the pelvic floor. INSTEpp.

Khalsa, S. S., Ainley, V., Adolphs, R., Cameron, O. G., Critchley, H. D., Davenport, P. W., Feinstein, J. S., Feusner, J. D., Garfinkel, S. N., Lane, R. D., Mehling, W. E., Meuret, A. E., Nemeroff, C. B., Oppenheimer, S., Petzschner, F. H., Pollatos, O., Rhudy, J. L., Schramm, L. P., Simmons, W. K., . . . Heller, A. (2018). Interoception and mental health: a roadmap. *Biological Psychiatry. Cognitive Neuroscience and Neuroimaging, 3*(6), 501–513.

Luders, E., Thompson, P. M., & Toga, A. W. (2010). The development of the corpus callosum in the healthy human brain. *The Journal of Neuroscience: The Official Journal of the Society for Neuroscience, 30*(33), 10985–10990.

Nair, S., Sagar, M., Sollers, J., Consedine, N., & Broadbent, E. (2015). Do slumped and upright postures affect stress responses? A randomized trial. *Health Psychology, 34*(6), 632–641.

Parker, S. J., Strath, S. J., & Swartz, A. M. (2008). Physical activity measurement in older adults: relationships with mental health. *Journal of Aging and Physical Activity, 16*(4), 369–380.

Schmitt, C. M., & Schoen, S. (2022). Interoception: A multi-sensory foundation of participation in daily life. *Frontiers in Neuroscience, 16,* Articles 875200.

Shapiro, F. (2012). *Getting past your past: Take control of your life with self-help techniques from EMDR therapy.* Rodale.

Todd, J., & Aspell, J. E. (2022). Mindfulness, Interoception, and the body. *Brain Sciences, 12*(6), 696.

van den Hout, M. A., & Engelhard, I. M. (2012). How does EMDR work? *Journal of Experimental Psychopathology, 3*(5), 724–738.

Vulliemoz, S., Raineteau, O., & Jabaudon, D. (2005). Reaching beyond the midline: why are human brains cross wired? *The Lancet. Neurology, 4*(2), 87–99.

Zieliński, G., Ginszt, M., Zawadka, M., Rutkowska, K., Podstawka, Z., Szkutnik, J., & Gawda, P. (2021). The relationship between stress and masticatory muscle activity in female students. *Journal of Clinical Medicine, 10*(16).

Chapter 7

Breath: A Resource of Regulation

Daphne is a forty-two-year-old woman who, above all, is a professional. She has been dedicated and strategic and enjoys the position and independence she experiences from her career. Though she is currently single, a man she had been dating for some months had recently become unpredictable and rough. She ended the relationship but not before the sleeping bear of her trauma history had woken up.

As a child, Daphne experienced profound neglect. She had been caring for herself since the age of five, sleeping at different neighbors' houses and getting food from them as well. As she tells her story, it is clear that Daphne remembers very little from her early years. Somehow, she went to school most of the time, until high school. She started missing so often that the state got involved, and Daphne entered foster care at the age of sixteen. "Thankfully, they were good people," she says, sharing how they provided practical support she had never had. She got through school, and they helped set her up with scholarships to attend college.

It was a new start for her, and she jumped into the full experience. She worked hard at her studies and did reasonably well. She made friends and went to parties. It was during her junior year of college that the partying began to "spiral out of control." On three separate occasions she was sexually assaulted, the last requiring hospitalization. During the summer between her junior and senior year, she recovered physically and refocused herself on her school and work. Since then, she has been dedicated to her career and it has paid off.

With the recent abusive relationship, traumatic memories of her childhood and college disrupted the composure she had held together. She had trouble sleeping, feeling like her brain and body couldn't settle. She found herself on the verge of panic in meetings at work. Even going to

DOI: 10.4324/9781003521945-10

the grocery store began to feel like a monumental challenge. She went to therapy, ready and willing to do the work to heal. Still, she knew it would take some time – and in the meantime needed to get back some stability in daily living.

Breathing became the practical key that unlocked access to improved functioning. She learned breathing patterns that regulated her body for sleep. She developed breathing skills that made going to the grocery store doable. She even learned breathing interventions that staved off panic and promoted her mental engagement in meetings again. For her, these were crucial lifelines that allowed some normalcy to be restored, while she did the longer, necessary work of recovering from her trauma.

THE NATURE OF BREATH

Much has been written on the breath. Some of it useful, some of it not. Some of it outdated, some of it on the cutting edge. The narrow focus at hand is to present you with effective, research-based, proven interventions that are available to you and every other human to bring real change. Breathing poorly may be to blame for limits in mental health. Learning to breathe well could herald renewed experiences of mental wellness.

The chapter on breath takes place just about halfway through the book, a breather in the middle of fifteen resources. It's fitting for us to pause, inhale and exhale. It's a process needing to be more intentional than just breathing. In a recent ongoing, cross-sectional health survey, the rates of respiratory discomfort among adults in the United States were notable, even beyond those with specific risk factors or diagnosed breathing problems. The result was a stated need to target the "poor state of respiratory health" across the board (Pleasants et al., 2022). As a society, we are woefully dilapidated when it comes to how we breathe. To tell someone or yourself to "just take a breath" may not be helpful. It may actually exacerbate the problem. There is reason to believe many may need to relearn how to breathe. When we do, we have within us, a sacrosanct and impervious power supporting mental wellness.

Before going further, I want to acknowledge what, for some, is an elephant in the room. To focus on breathing can require some to focus on their trauma. As a therapist primarily treating trauma, I have found it to be common for trauma survivors to develop less-than-optimal breathing patterns, and when they try to improve them, find that they are triggered or reminded of their trauma. It can be very troubling. Fear or terror can cause the body to instinctively hold the breath. Additionally, holding the breath can buffer the full force of painful feelings (Edwards, 2008). For reasons such as these, a person who has gone through trauma may associate holding the breath with survival. Even if the response is not as noticeable as breath holding, breathing patterns may shift in subtle ways in the course of surviving. When trying to correct or improve breathing, the signal that goes off in the brain indicates that the successful survival technique is being taken away along with safety. Perhaps you've experienced this, perhaps not. Suffice it to say, learning to breathe better, though crucial, may not be easy for you.

But it is necessary. It is worthy work to restore healthy breathing, creating improved patterns distinct from either a trauma history or from an ongoing lack of proper use. The territory of the breath is a birthright but requires maintenance with learning and practice. If you are one who finds your experience of trauma makes the work of breath seem daunting, I invite you to proceed slowly, but deliberately.

Breath is a regulating resource constantly present and within our immediate influence. Breath is one of the great universals, as each living person has some access to it. The access to the resource may differ person to person, but the important point is the degree to which we access what is available to us. At this moment, we all have breath.

However, as a modern culture, we are largely misusing the capacity to breathe. Chronically breathing breaths that are too shallow, too fast, and too ineffective contribute to lower brain functioning and mental health disruption (Pujari & Parvathisam, 2022). Improved breathing improves mental well-being. I have had clients refrain from meditation or approach breathing practices with trepidation because of health conditions that make breathing uncomfortable. It's an understandable reservation, but one that needs to be pushed against. Practices of breathing can improve mental health even with limitations due to disease; furthermore, practices of breathing can improve the problematic breathing conditions themselves (Nestor, 2020). The latter is beyond the scope of mental health. Our focus is going to zero in on ways that breath can positively influence mental wellness, and how we can harness that kind of breath.

Breath, Interoception, and the Nervous System

One way of using breath harkens back to a concept we've discussed throughout this work: interoception. Proper breathing can optimize interoceptive processes (Balban et al., 2023). The respiratory system is connected to the autonomic nervous system (ANS), the cardiovascular system, and the gastrointestinal system as well as the brain (Hamasaki, 2020). The interconnectedness of those particular systems provides data of our entire internal workings. The nature of the function of breathing means that we can read by our breath some of what interoception may provide us. Breath provides a way we can communicate directly and clearly with those systems, resulting in great influence over our mental wellness.

Speaking of the ANS, it is worth painting a brief picture of this system as relates to mental health and breathing because it is a key piece in how breathing is such a potent resource. The central nervous system (CNS) consists of two branches. One branch is called the sympathetic; it is the alarm response, or what's commonly considered responsible for the "fight-or-flight" response. It's "sympathetic" because it "feels with" other systems and stimuli. It is reactive, responding to irritants and stimulation. It arms the entire system to actively engage. The other branch is called the parasympathetic. It is meant to be the default posture of the central nervous system. It is where we "rest and digest" (Gibbons, 2019). The root "para" means "beside" or "beyond." It stands distinct from a reactionary connection to stimulus and events. If the nervous system were like a tree, then the parasympathetic would be the roots, deep and grounded, stable. The sympathetic would be the lofty branches, changing and responding to any type of wind.

When sympathetic activity is initiated by a perception of threat or stress, our entire system is ready to act. Basically, our systems are on their toes, ready to spring into action, which is very helpful when an action is needed. Unfortunately, for a myriad of reasons, there is a tendency to live day-to-day life with a degree of our sympathetic system activated as if it is our default mode. This is not how the CNS functions best. The parasympathetic is meant to be the resting condition, in which state we have more emotion regulation and control (Sturm et al., 2018). Gratefully, we are not at the mercy of our current patterns of response.

Get this: "Both arms of the autonomic nervous system are under the control of the central respiratory centres" (Russo, et al., 2017). We can pace either branch of the CNS with our breath, which although largely functions involuntarily, is absolutely under voluntary influence. By simply altering how we breathe, by breathing well, we can change our habituated or overworked sympathetic response. We can return to the intended default of a grounded parasympathetic posture.

Breathing Well

So what does it mean to breathe well? First of all, we should be breathing through our nose. The mouth is for eating, drinking, and talking; the nose is built for breathing. Nose breathing harvests more oxygen from the air, filters out harmful invaders, warms and moistens the air for optimal use. Nose breathing accomplishes things that mouth breathing cannot, perhaps most relevantly that it engages the parasympathetic system (Ruth, 2015).

All the practices we will learn about and attempt in this chapter are built on the essential foundation of inhaling through the nose.

Secondly, most people "over breathe," meaning we take in too many inefficient, shallow breaths, almost always through the mouth (Ruth, 2015). We are meant for fewer, longer breaths. Over time, learning to deepen the inhale and lengthen the exhale, and briefly extend the pause in between, has health ramifications for the entire human system (Tobe & Saito, 2020). Six breaths per minute is noted as optimal "slow" breathing for regular respiration, regulating the sympathetic and parasympathetic systems (Russo et al., 2017).

The basics of breathing well will not only lead to improved mental health regulation on a daily basis but can also offer powerful intervention. In leaving no stone unturned for mental health, we must consider the breath as "psychological studies have revealed breathing practice to be an effective non-pharmacological intervention for emotion enhancement, including a reduction in anxiety, depression, and stress" (Ma et al., 2017). As regular "slow" breathing through the nose can prepare the system to have a default parasympathetic state, specific breathing practices can train us to access the parasympathetic system or temper the sympathetic when threats arise. Our mental wellness, how we feel and function in any given moment, does not have to be reactive to the circumstances around us; we can be rooted in the parasympathetic calm through the influence of the breath. Controlled deep breathing reduces activity in the sympathetic nervous system, bringing balance with increased activation of the parasympathetic nervous system (Soni et al., 2015).

Breathing for Emotional and Cognitive Health

A single breathing practice positively influences blood pressure, heart rate, and oxygenation, which impact many systems, not the least of which are the systems that shape our mental health. Those who engage in ongoing breathing practices experience improved mental health (Ma et al., 2017). It's that simple. Both our processing of emotions and our cognitive processing are connected to breathing, by being intrinsically intertwined with the autonomic nervous system.

Often, people begin therapy because of problematic emotional or mental experiences. They feel a sadness beyond their capacity to cope. They feel angry in a way that is hard to control. They feel fear in the course of daily living. For emotions to be regulated by breathing is no small thing in the work of mental health. There are many effective, therapeutic interventions that aren't available to some of my clients for various reasons. Time and ability can be constraints. Some mental health interventions require a certain degree of mental capacity in order to attempt them. Not so with the breath. Any ability to breathe can lend itself to breathing practice, and therefore, emotional regulation and support (Pujari & Parvathisam, 2022). The positive impact of improved breathing on mental health is far-reaching, improving subtle daily functioning and more severe mental illness, inviting immediate change and long-term benefit (Ashhad et al., 2022).

Breathing practices also improve cognition. Less frequently do people come to my office saying they want to improve their cognition, yet more need it than they realize. Our cognition determines our perception of ourselves and the world around us, going beyond just our conscious thinking and including our sensory systems and higher processing (Soni et al., 2015). A daily regimen of simple, deep breathing practice has been clinically demonstrated to improve and maintain cognitive ability.

THE SCIENCE OF BREATH

The basic nature of breathing contributes to our neglect of the role it plays. The idea that breath, so commonplace and overused, could make a sizable difference in mental wellness may seem too obvious or simple to be true. I would argue that the very ordinariness of breathing is the very reason why it should be one of the first things we check when mental health seems off kilter. If I'm driving down the road and my car suddenly starts to lose steam, I check the gas gauge first. Even though I use it every single time I drive my car and it's the maintenance I provide for my car most regularly, it is because the car is so dependent on it that I will check that first. So it should be with mental health and the breath.

Consider the times when something seems off in your mental wellness: brain fog, toeing the line of inappropriate anger, fears like a dripping faucet, on the edge of panic, a background anxiety like ringing in the ears, or a growing gray restlessness. We are likely to not consider poor breathing as a serious source of the problem and so overlook it as a serious solution. Let's reconsider. As the breath is available to you now, and as it is intricately connected to your nervous system and mental health in general, let's examine ways a force so readily available could be applied for your mental wellness, even now.

Breath provides a direct line to mental health regulation through voluntary control of inhales and exhales. Though the breath can run on autopilot, thank goodness, we can also switch it over to manual and take control. Breathing, like many functions of the brain and body, is shaped through learning (Mckay et al., 2003). If you don't use a muscle, it will eventually atrophy. If you don't use a skill, you will likely lose your edge. If certain connections in the brain don't continue to fire and wire together, they will be "pruned." And yet, we can blaze new trails, creating new neural connections. Our brains and bodies have the capacity to be reworked. Muscles can be woken up and trained, skills can be honed, connections in the brain can be formed and strengthened.

Learning to Breathe Through the Nose

As noted, nose breathing is decidedly best for mental wellness. It is a key player in helping our nervous system default to the parasympathetic (rooted and calm). Nose breathing increases our capacity to respond to physiological symptoms of anxiety, balance mood, and regulate the "stress hormone" called cortisol (Balban et al., 2023). Breathing through the nose also brings an alignment between the olfactory centers of the brain with parts of the limbic system which houses the amygdala and hippocampus (Zelano et al., 2016). In other words, the parts of the brain associated with alarm as well as many of our intense emotions are supported by nasal breathing. We are more able to discern threats, incorporate memories, and regulate emotions with proper breathing.

Despite nasal breathing being the optimal breathing pattern for our human systems, a notable portion of humans habitually breathe through the mouth as a default (Lörinczi et al., 2024). How do we make a change? Thankfully, nasal breathing is one of those skills we can relearn and strengthen, making our instinctual breath a productive one. "Nasal breathing is self manifesting: performing it encourages subsequent ease" (Harbour et al., 2022). Our lack of nose breathing is largely due to lack of use. The more we practice, the more open, literally, the nasal passages become. It then follows that we have more access to engaging the parasympathetic nervous system (Ruth, 2015), strengthening the default posture of stability.

We relearn by practice. Repetition. Opportunity. As we increase awareness of the advantage of nose breathing, attention can be directed to breathing through the nose whenever we can. Spending even a minute with focused nose breathing can encourage the relearning. Additionally, specific training of our breathing has shown effectiveness in increasing proper breathing through the nose (Courtney et al., 2022), and in so doing benefits the whole human system.

Besides more mindful nasal breathing and intentional formal practices to encourage the same, some have utilized a process called "sleep taping" to encourage a shift out of mouth breathing. Essentially, "sleep taping" is sleeping with a small piece of medical tape holding the lips in a closed position. Though it encourages longer periods of relearning proper breathing and some have reported noticeable improvements with the practice, it does not have robust support in studies and it can pose some risk to certain populations (O'Halloran, 2024). It is worth consideration in consultation with health professionals.

Nose breathing is essential. With it, respiratory pathways are strengthened to reinforce the default parasympathetic state. Breathing properly improves our baseline of mental wellness while also serving as a go-to intervention. We can initiate specific patterns of breathing when we need them. The following regulating breathing practices are simple, yet effective in a wide variety of settings.

Slow Breath Response to Panic

The panic attack is a disruptive mental health experience. The hijacking that seems to take place of the whole system can be demoralizing, and it is exhausting. Fast acting antianxiety meds are broadly prescribed and are also addictive and habit-forming (Estrela et al., 2020). It's a common verbal response to someone having a panic attack to "just breathe," or "take a big breath." It seems the right response, but research tells a different story. Before a panic attack, people imperceptibly experience more rapid breathing (than even the already too-many-shallow breaths our society tends toward) and a decrease in carbon dioxide (Nestor, 2020). From a breathing perspective, these are dynamics that encourage physiological panic. Breath can be used to counter those trends. For my clients who struggle most with breathing related to panic or past trauma, focusing on learning to exhale more fully has been a productive place to start. Extending exhalations in comparison to inhalation is seen to reduce symptoms and frequency of panic (Van Diest et al., 2014). By breathing slower, less dramatic breaths, pausing in between inhale and exhale to allow the carbon dioxide to rise slightly to more optimal human level, panic attacks can be curbed or even stopped entirely.

Diaphragmatic Breathing

Next, a breathing practice called diaphragmatic breathing can be an effective response to "stress" (increased cortisol levels), to emotional dysregulation, and to difficulty focusing among other disruptions (Ma et al., 2017). To define what we're talking about, "diaphragmatic breathing is slow and deep breathing that affects the brain and cardiovascular, respiratory, and gastrointestinal systems through the modulation of autonomic nervous function" (Hamasaki, 2020). Movement of the diaphragm in breathing affects both the sympathetic and parasympathetic nervous systems, as well as improving activity of the nerves and brain. It's a breath pattern closer to what our natural, involuntary breath should ideally be, yet a bit more slow and deep. The introduction of attention to the diaphragm plays a part in managing connection with other systems in the body.

Mental distress does not occur in isolation in the brain. Often, in a moment of mental or emotional distress, we may not have the clarity to know the source of the distress. Diaphragmatic breathing is a great first defense, aligning and regulating our entire system (Hamasaki, 2020). The diaphragm is part of respiratory interoception, and connected to neural mechanisms that can regulate behavior and cognition (Chan et al., 2024). By initiating diaphragmatic breathing, we can support the system experiencing distress while also opening the lines of communication for interoception to better inform our response. When in doubt, engage in diaphragmatic breathing.

Physiological Sigh

The breath and its various rhythms are structured to work for us, but can become dysfunctional with lack of use. The sigh, also called the physiological sigh or cyclic sigh, is one of those rhythms too often in disrepair. As humans, we are meant to pace our breathing with deep sighs about every five minutes (Del Negro et al., 2018). It happens without notice, yet is important in refilling the lungs to refresh and keep active a greater portion of the lungs. Yet, as we've discussed, we are often only breathing with part of our lungs. Add to that, we are often functioning with an insidious and unidentified level of arousal in the sympathetic nervous system that is less likely to initiate that needed sigh. Physiological sighing is "characterized by deep breaths (two of them) followed by extended, relatively longer exhales, has been associated with psychological relief, shifts in autonomic states, and resetting of respiratory rate" (Balban et al., 2023). Due to the ease, accessibility, and effectiveness of the physiological sigh, it is a go-to practice that addresses real time mental duress. In a handful of moments, noticeable change can be secured.

The focus on these three types of voluntary breathwork among the many is intentional. They are available to everyone. They can be utilized without being observed by others. Together, they address most if not all mental health disruptions that may come up for you. They do not have to feel comfortable, easy, or enjoyable to be productive, like any practice or training. Once learned, they are easy to remember, repeat, and reestablish with your natural, intended breath.

BREATH IN PRACTICE

When we look to change something deeply ingrained or commonplace, the way forward requires intentional, consistent, technical practice. **We practice breath by learning to breathe better both as a default and as needed intervention.** We can overhaul our default modes, taking some time to push through the discomfort of change to produce new, beneficial patterns. As much of our breathing occurs involuntarily, the intensive work of restructuring the breath now becomes a long term investment.

Meditation Practice – A Guided Breathing Practice

Changing breath patterns requires attention and subtle changes. It may feel foreign or uncomfortable and at the same time calming and regulating. The following practice marks the way to return to what should be a normal, healthy breath, before moving a bit deeper into the beneficial diaphragmatic breath. It not only provides a practice space for relearning those breathing patterns, but also intentionally initiates mechanisms that bring about improved functioning, mood, and regulation. Go to kristaagler.com/book/keepinmind to listen to the provided audio or follow the accompanying prompts for a guided meditation on the healthy breath and the diaphragmatic breath.

Reflection Practice – Breath Observations

To fully reflect with awareness on your current relationship with breathing, consider pausing to follow the above guided practice before proceeding. Notice without placing judgment. The value of the breath is that it is available, matter-of-fact. Respond to the prompts in Table 7.1, observing your individual experience of breathing.

Conscious Practice – Comprehensive Breathing Practice Log

Commit to relearning more adaptive breathing patterns. Each day, practice four breathing exercises. Practice as needed, all at once, or spaced throughout each day. Refer to the brief descriptions to assist in your practice. Log your practice using Table 7.2 and at the end of the week, notice any changes you observe.

Table 7.1 Breath Observations

Prompt	Response
What is it like for you to pay attention to your breath?	
What parts are pleasant?	
What parts are unpleasant?	
Does illness, trauma, or other issues seem to be an obstacle to breathing for mental health? How so?	
Since breathing well is a learned skill, what is a next step you can take to continue improving the resource of your breath?	

Nose breathing – Set a timer for five minutes. Sit comfortably, yet naturally. Direct attention to inhaling and exhaling only through the nose for the duration of the practice. With the emphasis on nose breathing, don't alter your breathing rhythm at all. Don't slow or lengthen. Simply focus on the sensation and skill of inhaling and exhaling through the nose.

Exhaling in response to stress – After a stressful experience, or while recalling a stressful experience, focus on extending your exhale either through the nose or through the mouth. Be sure to inhale only through the nose, and focus on not only extending the exhale longer than the inhale but continue the exhale until the edge of comfort, just when you start to feel pressure. Then inhale through the nose. Repeat with a timer set for five minutes.

Diaphragmatic breath – Follow the provided guided meditation or practice independently as follows. Set a timer for five minutes. Lay down, placing one hand on the chest and one hand on the belly. Inhale through the nose deeply, causing the hand on the belly to rise first, perhaps the hand on the chest follows. Exhale slowly, allowing the hand on the belly to fall first, perhaps the hand on the chest follows. Repeat until the timer sounds.

Physiological sigh – Set a timer for just one or two minutes. Inhale through the nose deeply, and when you would naturally begin an exhale, take a second inhale again through the nose. This second inhale will likely be smaller than the first. Then release a controlled and complete exhale, slowly pressing all the air out through the mouth. Repeat until the timer goes off.

Lifestyle Practice – Physiological Sigh, Anytime

In day-to-day living, the physiological sigh may quickly become the most used, direct route to regulating your system. It is simple to use and brief

Table 7.2 *Comprehensive Breathing Practice Log*

	Nose Breathing	*Exhaling*	*Diaphragmatic*	*Sigh*
Sunday				
Monday				
Tuesday				
Wednesday				
Thursday				
Friday				
Saturday				

in its execution. You may find that exhaling through the nose is a bit more inconspicuous for use in more public contexts, allowing you to provide your brain and body with balance unnoticed by those around you. Remember, sighing is meant to be occurring in humans every five minutes. You may feel aware of it as you mindfully engage in the breath, but it will not be out of place or of notice to anyone around you. Mindfully nurture a reflexive response of shifting breathing patterns throughout the day, beginning with the physiological sigh.

IN SUMMARY

The resource of breath is constantly available and a skill that can be learned and relearned to improve cognitive function as well as emotional health. Through specific breathing practice, we can regulate the nervous system and tune into interoceptive messaging. Nose breathing is the optimal way of breathing and supports mental wellness. Our breathing patterns can be trained to function through the nose, to deepen and lengthen for holistic benefit. Extending exhales, diaphragmatic breathing, and the physiological sigh are three breathing patterns that can be widely used to support mental health in any context at any time.

We are breathing. We can learn to breathe better. Improved breathing improves mental health. May we not waste our breath.

REFERENCES

Ashhad, S., Kam, K., Del Negro, C. A., & Feldman, J. L. (2022). Breathing rhythm and pattern and their influence on emotion. *Annual Review of Neuroscience, 45*(1), 223–247.

Balban, M. Y., Neri, E., Kogon, M. M., Weed, L., Nouriani, B., Jo, B., Holl, G., Zeitzer, J. M., Spiegel, D., & Huberman, A. D. (2023). Brief structured respiration practices enhance mood and reduce physiological arousal. *Cell Reports. Medicine, 4*(1), Article 100895.

Chan, P. Y. S., Lee, L. Y., & Davenport, P. W. (2024). Neural mechanisms of respiratory interoception. *Autonomic Neuroscience*, Article 103181.

Courtney, R., Engel, R., Grace, S., Potts, A., Riordan, B., Ireland, K., & Sukhtankar, A. (2022). Functional nasal breathing rehabilitation: Effectiveness and feasibility of an online integrative breathing therapy protocol. *International Journal of Orofacial Myology and Myofunctional Therapy, 48*(1), 1–14.

Del Negro, C. A., Funk, G. D., & Feldman, J. L. (2018). Breathing matters. *Nature Reviews. Neuroscience, 19*(6), 351–367.

Edwards, S. D. (2008). Breath psychology: fundamentals and applications. *Psychology and Developing Societies, 20*(2), 131–164.

Estrela, M., Herdeiro, M. T., Ferreira, P. L., & Roque, F. (2020). The use of antidepressants, anxiolytics, sedatives and hypnotics in europe: focusing on mental health care in portugal and prescribing in older patients. *International Journal of Environmental Research and Public Health, 17*(22).

Gibbons, C. H. (2019). Basics of autonomic nervous system function. *Handbook of clinical neurology, 160*, 407–418.

Hamasaki, H. (2020). Effects of diaphragmatic breathing on health: a narrative review. *Medicines (Basel), 7*(10).

Harbour, E., Stöggl, T., Schwameder, H., & Finkenzeller, T. (2022). Breath tools: a synthesis of evidence-based breathing strategies to enhance human running. *Frontiers in Physiology, 13*, Article 813243.

Lörinczi, F., Vanderka, M., Lörincziová, D., & Kushkestani, M. (2024). Nose vs. mouth breathing–acute effect of different breathing regimens on muscular endurance. *BMC Sports Science, Medicine and Rehabilitation, 16*(1), 42.

Ma, X., Yue, Z.-Q., Gong, Z.-Q., Zhang, H., Duan, N.-Y., Shi, Y.-T., Wei, G.-X., & Li, Y.-F. (2017). The effect of diaphragmatic breathing on attention, negative affect and stress in healthy adults. *Frontiers in Psychology, 8*.

Mckay, L. C., Evans, K. C., Frackowiak, R. S., & Corfield, D. R. (2003). Neural correlates of voluntary breathing in humans. *Journal of Applied Physiology, 95*(3), 1170–1178.

Nestor, J. (2020). *Breath: The New Science of a Lost Art.* Penguin Life.

O'Halloran, K. D. (2024). Mouth taping: a little less conversation, a little more action, please! *The Journal of Physiology, 602*(15), 3605–3607.

Pleasants, R. A., Heidari, K., Ohar, J., Donohue, J. F., Lugogo, N. L., Kanotra, S. M., Kraft, M., Mannino, D. M., & Strange, C. B. (2022). Respiratory Symptoms among US Adults: a Cross-Sectional Health Survey Study. *Pulmonary Therapy, 8*(3), 255–268.

Pujari, V., & Parvathisam, S. (2022). Breathing Your Way To Better Brain Function: The Role Of Respiration In Cognitive Performance. *Journal of Pharmaceutical Negative Results*, 8214–8219.

Russo, M. A., Santarelli, D. M., & O'Rourke, D. (2017). The physiological effects of slow breathing in the healthy human. *Breathe, 13*(4), 298–309.

Ruth, A. (2015). The health benefits of nose breathing. *Nursing in General Practice.*

Soni, S., Joshi, L. N., & Datta, A. (2015). Effect of controlled deep breathing on psychomotor and higher mental functions in normal individuals. *Indian Journal of Physiology and Pharmacology, 59*(1), 41–7.

Sturm, V. E., Sible, I. J., Datta, S., Hua, A. Y., Perry, D. C., Kramer, J. H., . . . & Rosen, H. J. (2018). Resting parasympathetic dysfunction predicts prosocial helping deficits in behavioral variant frontotemporal dementia. *Cortex, 109*, 141–155.

Tobe, M., & Saito, S. (2020). Analogy between classical Yoga/Zen breathing and modern clinical respiratory therapy. *Journal of Anesthesia, 34*(6), 944–949.

Van Diest, I., Verstappen, K., Aubert, A. E., Widjaja, D., Vansteenwegen, D., & Vlemincx, E. (2014). Inhalation/exhalation ratio modulates the effect of slow breathing on heart rate variability and relaxation. *Applied Psychophysiology and Biofeedback*, *39*, 171–180.

Zelano, C., Jiang, H., Zhou, G., Arora, N., Schuele, S., Rosenow, J., & Gottfried, J. A. (2016). Nasal Respiration Entrains Human Limbic Oscillations and Modulates Cognitive Function. *The Journal of Neuroscience: The Official Journal of the Society for Neuroscience*, *36*(49), 12448–12467.

Chapter 8

Water: A Resource of Hydration, Proximity, and Contact

Rachel finally went to therapy in "maddening levels of pain." She had lost a child when he was just two years old. The grief was pain run wild, and it brought back the hurt she experienced in the twenty-seven years prior to her loss. She had grown up in a "cultlike" context, in which she recalled abuse and psychological confusion. Although she was out of all that and by all observable standards had "made a good life for herself," the death of her son "put a magnifying glass over all that's been wrong." She likened her internal suffering to "being split in two yet everyone watching acts like it's not happening." Feeling crazy, she had urges to run away from her husband, their four-year-old daughter, and indeed, all of life.

She couldn't imagine therapy could help as she could hardly imagine getting out of bed another day. She listened quietly as the therapist laid out the steps they would eventually take and became offended when the only suggestion given in the first session was to increase her water intake. It felt disproportionately small to the level of anguish she had surely clearly communicated. Seeing her face, the therapist responded, "We need to start slow. Very slow. Water will help your brain do all that comes next."

Mainly because she didn't know what else to do, Rachel started drinking more water. Especially when she felt the urge to run away. Although she would say it didn't make her feel better, she would say it helped her feel different. At that point, different was a good place to start. Of course Rachel had a longer journey to go. She moved forward slowly but surely. Water wasn't the solution, but it was a key partner that went with her.

DOI: 10.4324/9781003521945-11

THE NATURE OF WATER

For mental health, we find water to be essential and functional in ways that go beyond drinking ounces for basic survival. There are a few touchpoints of where water impacts mental health, some of it subtle, and some of it startling. Whether we're drinking it, swimming in it, or observing it, water helps the brain function better. **Water is a versatile resource, bringing balance through internal and external means of neural regulation.**

Water: Crucial, Practical, Effective

Right out of the gate, it should be clear that the role of water in mental health is central. For example, one of the most widely reported experiences of mental distress can be caused, aggravated, or improved directly by your level of hydration. Anxiety consists of, among other things, a learned pathway connecting neurotransmitter signaling with environmental experience (Martin et al., 2009). Once someone has experienced significant anxiety or panic, a neural connection is formed. The more anxiety is experienced, the stronger that connection grows. Dehydration plays into that.

Symptoms of dehydration parallel many symptoms of anxiety: fatigue, confusion, difficulty breathing, dizziness, dry mouth, changes in heart rate. There are causal and correlative components to that relationship. For one, dehydration contributes to higher levels of anxiety (Ganio et al., 2011). For another, as anxiety is in part a learned neural circuit making sense of various stimuli (Calhoon & Tye, 2015), the more frequently the brain is dehydrated, the more connections are established with anxiety, perpetuating the problem. Dehydration, just by manifesting similar symptoms can initiate or intensify anxiety. If we have chronic dehydration, there can be a constant launching of that learned anxiety response. Just as dehydration can trigger anxiety, hydration can mitigate it.

Connecting, or reconnecting, to drinking water seems an easy, necessary, and such a practical place to start. And yet, drinking water for mental health is only one facet of the role it can play in mental well-being. At the surface, there may not be much surprise at the integral nature of water in our health in general. Throughout time, entire cultures have congregated around water or shaped their way of being around their relationship to it (Anderson et al., 2019). The majority of life on the planet depends on water for survival. Water is ubiquitous, so it may be tempting to think, "Drink water. Check. Let's move on." I invite you to tune in, refresh your current appreciation of water, and see what else it has to offer.

Our pursuit of mental health should be practical above all things. In my clinical observation, the feedback from clients regarding water interventions has been pretty profound. It has not been a panacea by any means, but for something simple to be directly effective is welcomed relief to those suffering. For something available to be immediately useful is heartening.

More than Hydration

Although hydration is key, there are other ways water supports mental health. Beyond drinking water, proximity to it brings about marked improvement. From splashing in the shallows to full immersion, from standing shoreside to hearing the rain on the roof, the brain seems to respond to a wide variety of interactions with water in ways that are beneficial.

If you've been to the ocean or stood by a river or even gotten caught in a rainstorm, you can probably attest to the mental shift that can happen around water. The properties of the movement of water and the way light and sound bounces off it creates an environment for which the brain has an affinity (Nichols, 2014). Research reveals that there are healing effects by being in a water environment. Being around bodies of water not only reduces tension and symptoms of physiological stress but it also provokes uplifted states of emotion (Tang et al., 2024). The regulation and functioning of the brain are served by being near water. The positive effect of water is not just limited to oceans, rivers, and lakes. The visual, auditory, and sensorimotor experiences with water also hold influence in smaller capacities, even with water we encounter indoors (Ting & Bahauddin, 2022). To be in the presence of water is to have a resource for mental well-being – if approached intentionally and mindfully.

Taking it to another level, there are mental health benefits to actually coming into contact with water. These benefits are being recognized and ways of using water for treatment are increasing in popularity. Water activities have been seen to aid in the relief of PTSD for veterans with a "prescription"-like effect (Nichols, 2014). Even in office settings for therapy, when using sensory or tactiles interventions, we refer to "dry mediums" or "wet mediums." The former hold their own shape, the latter take the shape of their container. So dry mediums would include rocks, marbles, things of that nature. Wet mediums include sand, clay, and of course water. Dry mediums tend to be grounding, while wet mediums can help activate, bring movement, or relieve "stuckness," working from the base of the brain through the limbic system, aiding in the processing of difficult content (O'Connor et al., 2015). And so water, by being both a wet medium bringing activation to the limbic system as well as an environmental element assisting the brain in optimal functioning, is a unique and potent resource for mental health support. It aids in psychological reflection while also supporting the brain mechanistically. Water invites deeper processing and adaptive growth while also coming alongside your brain to regulate and soothe. Any water you're around is a resource for your mental health: the shower, the thunderstorm, the tepid water as you wash your hands. The power is not in the size, strength, or novelty we often appreciate in large bodies of water. The power is in the manner in which we come to the water available to us.

THE SCIENCE OF WATER

Addressing water directly, Antoine de Saint-Exupéry said, "not necessary to life, but rather life itself, thou fillest us with a gratification that exceeds the delight of the senses" (Saint-Exupéry et al., 1940). In similar wonder, it's been said that "water is H2O, hydrogen two parts, oxygen one, but there is also a third thing, that makes it water, and nobody knows what it is" (Lawrence, 1930). At first glance, it's not straightforward what about water makes it so useful. It doesn't take much searching to find the evidence of its utility. As we survey some of the science involved in how water supports mental wellness, we will find that the many properties of water can be strategically applied to create change throughout the brain-body system. **Water provides us with an immediate, tangible pipeline to the neurological, physical, and psychological aspects of mental health.**

Hydration and Mental Health

You are composed mainly of water. It is estimated that the human body is between 45% and 75% water (Garcia et al., 2019). These numbers vary between studies and are based on age and gender of a person. The brain has a slightly higher concentration of water at approximately 80% (Oros-Peusquens et al., 2019). It is part of our physiological makeup and functions within us as an essential nutrient. Without water, we die. Without enough water, we start to break down physically and mentally. It is nonnegotiable.

Mild dehydration can impact attention, psychomotor and regulatory functions, thought, memory, perception, reaction times, alertness, concentration, fatigue, and anxiety. The relationship is established. It's also estimated that potentially 75% of adults in America are chronically dehydrated (Cohen and Bria, 2018). With that high of a rate, and the high rate of the symptoms listed above, it's not over the top or superfluous to emphasize: we need to hydrate (Wilson and Morley, 2003).

Now, we don't just do that by drinking water, though that is a simple and great place to start. There's an often-quoted stat that we should aim to drink half our body weight in ounces. So, if you weigh 200 pounds, you should drink 100 ounces of water, or so goes the theory. In actuality, this statistic originated in a study in which hydration through food contributed to the targeted amount of ounces (Cohen and Bria, 2018). Our hydration doesn't just come from water. I highlight the fact not to discourage you from drinking water, but to shift the perspective that hydration is more nuanced and perhaps more accessible than constant guzzling. By improving our understanding of water, we may utilize it more effectively and avoid counterproductive overuse.

According to Dr. Joseph G. Verbalis with Georgetown University, the kidneys can release a quart of fluid each hour. More than that overwhelms the kidneys, and can lead to unhealthy water retention (2022). It's possible to have too much of a good thing (Cohen and Bria, 2018), which is why the recommendation is not to chug as much water as you can throughout the day. Verbalis suggests drinking when you're thirsty, unless specifics of your situation would indicate otherwise.

In my clinical observation, along with statistics mentioned above, I have seen that awareness of thirst is not a given. The skill of interoception, when it comes to thirst and hydration, often needs nurturing. It may take some practice to identify thirst accurately. The more foods we consume with added sugar or saturated fat, we decrease our interoceptive sensitivity to thirst (Brannigan et al., 2015). Perhaps you have heard the advice to drink water when you feel hungry, which comes from this interoceptive confusion when thirst is veiled, mistaken for hunger.

Careful observation of thoughts, emotions, and body sensations before and after a drink of water will begin to strengthen interoceptive attention to the whole-body experience of being hydrated. Lacking the discernment of being dehydrated is a liability to mental wellness.

Optimizing Hydration for Mental Health

There is a constant ebb and flow to hydration, but it's not as simple as water in, water out. There is perpetual movement with water, flowing with directional purpose. There is coherence in the way of water, how it falls, saturates, and evaporates. The engagement of our bodies with water, both how it hydrates and how we expel moisture, follows patterns as well. The better we understand these trends, the more we improve our relationship with water. Having a clearer understanding of how our bodies actually handle hydration is an important springboard into full use of the resource.

Water is widely known to have three forms: ice, liquid, and vapor. It may be less well known that it can also present in a slightly gel-like state. The slight change in structure isn't always observable, but it presents at a cellular level. Our cells mimic this more structured, gel-like form of water (Pollack, 2003). This type of water is often referred to as structured water. Our body at a cellular level favors water in that gel-like state, making hydration more effective. In this slightly different structure, water not only helps the body hold moisture more efficiently, it becomes a better conductor, improving the body's use of electrolytes and minerals (Cohen and Bria, 2018). As the water in plants often presents in such a gel-like structure, adding citrus juice or cucumber slices to water, or even just eating an apple alongside a drink of water can optimize the conditions for hydration.

Every day we do things that draw out our water that have dehydrating properties. That's part of living. The goal is not to stop any activity that costs water, but the goal is to be mindful of it and draw a conscious connection with those activities and the impact it may have on our mental health, adjusting water intake accordingly. The goal is awareness and response, not a hard-set list of rules. It will look different for each person.

Being mindful of the impact water has on our mental health as it hydrates our body and brain is also a regulatory practice. It encourages that skill of interoception necessary for adaptive mental health responses. Paying attention to our internal senses positively influences mental health in regular day-to-day functioning. Having that additional awareness and attuned senses through whole-body engagement enhances the enjoyment as well as utilization of water.

Benefits of Being Around Water

In looking for ways to improve mental health with what is available to us, one consideration is where we are in physical location. For the same reasons we pursue water destinations for vacations or find waterfront properties more desirable, putting ourselves near water is a move to improve mental health. "Studies have indicated that waterscapes can play an important therapeutic role in the physical, mental, and social health of residents, by lowering psychological distress" (Zhang et al., 2021). Waterscapes include any physical surrounding that has a prominent water feature from a fountain, river, lake, and so forth. They can be naturally occurring or designed.

Some even advocate for a focus on developing waterscapes in urban contexts in order to provide mental health support to the masses. Cities with canals or rivers within the concrete jungle provide their residents with improved mental health, more balanced mood, decreased anxiety, and even reduction of psychotic symptoms (Bergou et al., 2022). Being creaturess of motion and migration, we have the ability to intentionally place ourselves near water from time to time, whether it be the beach, a small nearby river, or a large fountain at the local mall. Though seemingly artificial, studies of mental health and water indicate similar positive effects when even just looking at images or videography of water as when we're around the real thing (Nichols, 2014).

The benefits of proximity to water are due in part to the way water changes the sensory input. Water features impact sounds, reducing chaotic or competing noise. It also provides a softening reflection of light making visual input more favorable. Many of our sensory perceptions are positively altered by the presence of water. When humans have regular nearness to waterscapes, they have a reported improved psychological wellness, more robust resilience, enhanced emotional release, and heightened cognitive performance (Zhang et al., 2021). For centuries the poets have appreciated what research continues to demonstrate: the beauty of water is not superficial, but transformative. As Wendell Berry said, "I come into the presence of still water, and I feel above me the day-blind stars waiting for their light. For a time I rest in the grace of the world, and am free" (1995).

Benefits of Contact With Water

So far in our exploration of the human affinity for mental health, we've explored ways that the brain and body work together, and that all our senses from the external to the internal have a role to play in taking greater care of our minds.

Among the foundational elements, water can far and away play the most beneficial role in keeping us "in touch" with the sensory world. It has a tangible quality, a weight, heavier than air – yet unlike earth – we can move through it (Nichols, 2014).

As humans, our compatibility with water is functional. Our senses require it, are soothed by it. It activates and grounds our systems from the point of contact with skin to our nerves and everything in between. Water is not merely an essential nutrient or a favorable environment, though it is those things. From the moment of any contact with water, the skin initiates messaging between sensory inputs and neural reception (Filingeri & Ackerley, 2017). Water also contains properties that synergistically connect the various human systems at play in mental health, and accesses them through the sophisticated sensory systems. Water is not an additive; it is a catalyst.

Beyond the benefit of hydration or of environmental relief, actual contact or immersion in water has its own remedial work to do for mental health. For mental health (and physical health for that matter), entire therapies have been developed upon the research of the benefits of being in water. “Recent studies have assessed the psychological effects of hydrotherapy, such as mental relaxation, mental fatigue, quality of life, and depression/stress” (Kelly & Bird, 2022).

When our bodies are immersed, the blood flow within our bodies behaves differently. It shifts from the limbs to be more concentrated near the heart. Circulation within the muscles increases. Immersion impacts many systems throughout the body, while improving cognition, memory, and trauma-recovery at a brain level (Becker et al., 2009). The density of water surrounding the body when it is immersed complements the density of the water, making up 60% of our bodies. It creates a regulating sensation, and the buoyancy created alleviates the pressure of gravity on our systems (An et al., 2019). These effects are specific to immersion when a large portion of the body is submerged under water. There are also effects of water on the body based on temperature, through immersion or with similar effect through nonimmersive contact, like a shower.

Generally speaking, warm water immersion can support the cardiovascular system, while cold immersion can serve the neuromuscular system (An et al., 2019). Cold-water immersion can encourage a positive mood state, give an elevated experience of well-being, support people with mood disorders, disrupt anxiety patterns, and have a positive influence on a slew of neurotransmitters (Yankouskaya et al., 2023). Even with these benefits, it is noted that cold immersion can increase activity in the sympathetic nervous system, potentially having adverse implications for those prone to anxiety. Alternatively, warm water immersion is seen to affect the nervous system similar to meditation, bringing the system into parasympathetic grounding and regulation (Becker et al., 2009).

Though various forms of research will point to specific ways of coming into contact with water that are optimal, what's most important is using what is available to you. You may not have ready access to the cold Pacific Ocean or a hot tub, but you may have access to a hot shower or a brief walk in the cold rain. The best support for your mental wellness is in using what is around you, within reach, and in doing so knowing that a marginal difference is still improvement.

WATER IN PRACTICE

We can hydrate, we can notice the water around us, and we can move with and immerse in water, all for therapeutic effect. We are dependent on water. We absolutely need water to function, and yet it holds, beyond its basic utility, a multipurpose usefulness that in actual fact alters our mental state. **We put water into practice through mindful consumption, observation, and interaction.**

Meditation Practice – A guided Meditation for Drinking Water

The simple act of drinking water can serve our mental health by hydration and also through contact. By engaging in the process mindfully, employing interoception with slow, deliberate attention, we can gain even more from the experience. Go to kristaagler.com/book/keepinmind to listen to the provided audio or follow the accompanying prompts for a guided meditation for drinking water.

Reflection Practice – Cultivate Awareness of Water: Hydration and Contact

Even if you have good water habits, strengthening awareness is valuable work, especially as it relates to mental health. At this time, the goal is not about changing your water intake; the goal is to reflect. It is about drawing a connection with hydration and its potential impact on your mental health, equipping you for a faster response time. Fatigue and brain fog can be some telltale indicators of a need for hydration, a sign of thirst (Cohen and Bria, 2018). Acknowledge the relationship dehydration may have with your mental health, and gently notice any correlations your mental health may have with dehydrating food, drink, or activities. Similarly, when you drink water, notice any relief or improvement that becomes available. Begin considering how to support your mental health hydration in awareness.

Many of our daily opportunities to make contact with water are connected with mundane activities of daily living: showering, brushing teeth, making tea or coffee, driving in the rain, and so forth. Repetition can ease the effort of an action and reduce required attention, leaving us going through the motions and missing out on benefits that come with mindfulness. Beyond the commonplace, perhaps you have ready opportunities for water hobbies or to be around natural waterscapes. Perhaps even such leisure activities have lost their impact due to frequency. Attention applied in new ways encourages new neural connections between what we observe and the potentially powerful effects demonstrated in research. Use Table 8.1 and reflect.

Table 8.1 *Awareness of Water*

Prompt	Response
What signals specific to you indicate that you are thirsty? What are your thoughts on hydration and your mental health? What could improve your use of hydration for mental health?	
Identify one time to mindfully and intentionally hydrate during your day.	
When do you interact with water throughout the day? How do you experience these interactions? What could make your interactions with water more mindful and intentional?	
Identify one daily opportunity you have to mindfully come into contact with water?	

Daily incidents of hydration or contact with water are opportunities to invest in your mental health. These motions you're already taking, altered slightly with purpose, become active participants in your mental wellness.

Conscious Practice - Sensory and Interoceptive Water Practice

Write down the times you make contact with water during a regular week: showering, brushing teeth, washing hands, doing dishes, bathing your kids, intentional hydrating, watering plants, and so forth. For one week, focus on using all of your senses when engaging in these activities.

Now, as you're engaging in the activity, cycle your attention through the five exteroceptive senses: sight, sound, smell, touch, and taste. Keep cycling through. Then, either subsequently or alternatively, engage that growing skill of interoception to notice internal sensations changing as you engage in that act of contact with water. This practice develops and strengthens a connection between mindful attention and the regulating properties of water in as many places as you make contact with it.

Lifestyle Practice – A Lifestyle Connected to Water

Through hydration, observation, and exposure, beginning to connect all our interactions with water with our mental wellness improves a symbiotic relationship that is inherent to being human. Attention bias, that phenomenon of noticing more instances of a thing we're already thinking about, can work in our favor. With water on our minds, we can be more highly attuned to the opportunities water affords us to address mental health needs.

Read through the list in Table 8.2 of potential interactions with water. As you go through your day and your week, notice or initiate experiences with them. Use the provided space to note any observations of the effects of water on well-being.

IN SUMMARY

If how you drink water and notice water around you becomes a conscious aspect of your mental health lifestyle, you will almost constantly be making positive investments in your mental wellness. Water is prevalent in most of our day-to-day lives, and so the challenge is to engage with the resource with mindful attention and to actually utilize it for hydration, observation, and contact. From initial sensory contact to the deep regulation of the nervous system, from hydration to the positive effects of water in our immediate environment, water works with our brain and serves our mental wellness.

That being said, there are far too many places in the world where water is not easily accessed. As extensive as waterways and plumbing can seem, it's not a given that all have access to clean drinking water. The goal of this book is to highlight resources that are as widely available as possible, and as I write about water, there is an ever-present awareness that access is not a given.

Collectively, I want to draw our attention to the capacity we have to share our surplus of water with people and places that are truly thirsty. It may begin by giving a cup of cold water or having some extra bottles of water nearby in case you cross paths with someone who could use a drink. Because of what water does, such a simple act could begin to support the mental health of those right around you. Then perhaps look to your own community, to where you may have influence to improve the water availability in your own city or town. And then look beyond to where you could help make the vital and mental-health-invigorating resource of water available to others.

Table 8.2 *A Lifestyle Connected to Water*

Hydration	
Start the day hydrating your body with a good sized drink. Notice how your body responds.	
Intentionally notice thirst, and respond promptly with a drink of cold water.	
When experiencing mental disruption of any kind, respond with a drink of water.	
Hydrate using the gel-like form of water by adding citrus or cucumber to water.	
Pair hydration with gentle movement such as stretching or a short, slow walk.	
Drink slowly, consciously, and mindfully.	
Proximity/Contact	
For one day, choose a commute route that takes you by waterscapes.	
Immerse most of your body where available, whether the ocean, the local pool, or a bath.	
Mindfully make contact with uncomfortably (not painfully) cold water.	
Mindfully make contact with warm water.	
Seek out waterscapes in art or media.	

> The air, the water, and the ground are free gifts to humans, and no one has the power to portion them out in parcels. People must drink, breathe, and walk – and therefore each has a right to his share of earth. (Cooper, 1950)

Here's to water, and the share meant for each one of us.

REFERENCES

Anderson, E. P., Jackson, S., Tharme, R. E., Douglas, M., Flotemersch, J. E., Zwarteveen, M., Lokgariwar, C., Montoya, M., Wali, A., Tipa, G. T., Jardine, T. D., Olden, J. D., Cheng, L., Conallin, J., Cosens, B., Dickens, C., Garrick, D., Groenfeldt, D., Kabogo, J., . . . Arthington, A. H. (2019). Understanding rivers and their social relations: a critical step to advance environmental water management. *International Water Management Institute.*

Becker, B. E., Hildenbrand, K., Whitcomb, R. K., & Sanders, J. P. (2009). Biophysiologic effects of warm water immersion. *International Journal of Aquatic Research and Education, 3*(1), 4.

Bergou, N., Hammoud, R., Smythe, M., Gibbons, J., Davidson, N., Tognin, S., Reeves, G., Shepherd, J., Mechelli, A., & Clarke, T.-K. (2022). The mental health benefits of visiting canals and rivers: an ecological momentary assessment study. *Plos One, 17*(8).

Berry, W. (1995). *Openings: Poems.* Harcourt.

Brannigan, M., Stevenson, R. J., & Francis, H. (2015). Thirst interoception and its relationship to a Western-style diet. *Physiology & Behavior, 139,* 423–429.

Calhoon, G. G., & Tye, K. M. (2015). Resolving the neural circuits of anxiety. *Nature Neuroscience, 18*(10), 1394–1404.

Cohen, D., & Bria, G. (2018). *Quench: Beat fatigue, drop weight, and heal your body through the new science of optimum hydration.* Hachette.

Cooper, J. F. (1950). *The prairie.* Rinehart.

Filingeri, D., & Ackerley, R. (2017). The biology of skin wetness perception and its implications in manual function and for reproducing complex somatosensory signals in neuroprosthetics. *Journal of Neurophysiology, 117*(4), 1761–1775.

Ganio, M. S., Armstrong, L. E., Casa, D. J., McDermott, B. P., Lee, E. C., Yamamoto, L. M., Marzano, S., Lopez, R. M., Jimenez, L., Le Bellego, L., Chevillotte, E., & Lieberman, H. R. (2011). Mild dehydration impairs cognitive performance and mood of men. *The British Journal of Nutrition, 106*(10), 1535–1543.

Garcia, A. I. L., Morais-Moreno, C., Samaniego-Vaesken, M. L., Puga, A. M., Partearroyo, T., & Varela-Moreiras, G. (2019). Influence of water intake and balance on body composition in healthy young adults from spain. *Nutrients, 11*(8).

Kelly, J. S. & Bird, E. L. (2022). Improved mood following a single immersion in cold water. *Lifestyle Medicine, 3*(1).

Lawrence, D. H. (1930). *Pansies: Poems by D.H. Lawrence.* Secker.

Martin, E. I., Ressler, K. J., Binder, E., & Nemeroff, C. B. (2009). The neurobiology of anxiety disorders: brain imaging, genetics, and psychoneuroendocrinology. *The Psychiatric Clinics of North America, 32*(3), 549–575.

Nichols, W. J. (2014). *Blue Mind: The suprising science that shows how being near, in, on, or under water can make you happier, healthier, more connected, and better at what you do.* Back Bay Books.

O'Connor, K. J., Schaefer, C. E., & Braverman, L. D. (Eds.). (2015). *Handbook of play therapy* (2nd ed.). John Wiley & Sons.

Oros-Peusquens, A.-M., Loucao, R., Abbas, Z., Gras, V., Zimmermann, M., & Shah, N. J. (2019). A single-scan, rapid whole-brain protocol for quantitative water content mapping with neurobiological implications. *Frontiers in Neurology, 10.*

Pollack, G. H. (2003). The role of aqueous interfaces in the cell. *Advances in Colloid and Interface Science, 103*(2), 173–196.

Saint-Exupéry, A.d., Lewis, G. & Cosgrave, J. O. H. (1940). *Wind, sand and stars.* Harcourt, Brace & World.

Tang, H. F., Lee, A. Y., & Hung, S. H. (2024). Does built environment and natural leisure settings with bodies of water improve human psychological and physiological health? *Landscape and Ecological Engineering,* 1–12.

Ting, H. Y., & Bahauddin, A. (2022). The impact of blue space in the interior on mental health. *ARTEKS: Jurnal Teknik Arsitektur,* 7(1), 53–60.

Verbalis, J.G. (2022, October 24). Ask a doctor: What happens if I drink too much water? *The Washington Post.*

Wilson, M.M. G., & Morley, J. E. (2003). Impaired cognitive function and mental performance in mild dehydration. *European Journal of Clinical Nutrition, 57,* 24–9.

Zhang, X., Zhang, Y., Zhai, J., Wu, Y., & Mao, A. (2021). Waterscapes for Promoting Mental Health in the General Population. *International Journal of Environmental Research and Public Health, 18*(22), Article 11792.

Chapter 9

Provision: A Resource of the Approach to Nourishment

Alice went to therapy to address anxiety and depression rooted in a long history of being abused. Her abuse began with an uncle, then a cousin, then a boyfriend, then a first husband, and then a second husband. Alice was small and looked older than her years. Her demeanor was rough, but her words and perspective were uncommonly kind. She was working hard to provide for herself, her daughter, and her current boyfriend. Work was difficult due to her anxiety. Even so, she enjoyed her work delivering pizzas. She liked that most of the time she was driving her car that she had paid for herself. However, going to different locations every time and never knowing who would answer the door kept her body in an alarm state most of her shift.

During her first marriage, she had been addicted to pills, particularly benzodiazepines, so she wanted to find ways to get through the workday without medication. She had learned some regulation practices in therapy and was working with her therapist to find ways to initiate that learned calm using the sense of smell. The goal was to pair deep breathing and muscle relaxation with a smell that she could encounter by control at work. The therapist suggested aromatherapy. Alice suggested orange soda. For a week, she would practice daily getting to a place of relaxation, and then she would open a cold can of orange soda and inhale, smelling the vapor coming off the freshly agitated carbonation. Then she would take a sip, and exhale deeply. She took the skill on the job with her. The effect was beautiful. She was able, with that resource, to teach her brain to calm even in unknown situations at work. The benefit was not in the orange soda. It was in how she mindfully presented it to herself in response to a need. She was drawing from the resource of provision, of how we consume the nourishment available.

DOI: 10.4324/9781003521945-12

Unlike Alice, Kendrick would say he had an uneventful childhood and intact family life. He had worked at the library for almost 17 years, moving around most of his shift among the stacks of books. Despite the seeming stability in his life, the general wear and tear of the years resulted in a constant, low bubbling of anxiety. He was proactive in self-reflection and seeking out solutions, yet his wheels always seemed to be spinning.

In recent years, the anxiety began peaking at work, and it was typically worse in the morning. It seemed inexplicable, and he tried to ignore it, until an incident of passing out forced him to address it. He met with a clinician who evaluated his environment, potential triggers, and eventually his diet. It was fairly pristine: organic, variety of fruits and vegetables, very intentional. Still, things weren't adding up with the predictable cycle of his anxiety. The questions became more specific, inquiring what times of day he ate. He shared that he didn't eat breakfast and that his first meal of the day was at lunch around 1:00 p.m. A friend of his benefited from a fasting practice, and so he had been doing it for a couple years as well. He would drink coffee in the morning and then wait to eat until his lunch break.

He was eating all the "right" things, but was withholding them from his body when his body needed them. He was even ignoring signals his body had been sending like feeling lightheaded when going up stairs or feeling shaky. He attributed these symptoms to anxiety and never considered that his anxiety could be connected to how he was eating. With this awareness, he made changes, exploring what eating patterns worked best for his body. He discovered he did better with protein at breakfast before leaving for work, and often benefited from a snack midmorning, both before the time he was consuming his first calories previously. His "anxiety" symptoms plummeted, though he wondered how much of his experience was anxiety and how much was his body's hunger cues. Both were improved by a better use of provision, of changing how, not what, he ate.

THE NATURE OF PROVISION

The word "provision" can refer to food at a general level. However, it can also refer to the act or process of providing food, the act or process of providing nourishment. In considering provision as a resource for mental health, we are not just talking about food, but about the act and process of providing nourishment to our human system. So the resource of provision is not just about what you eat, but the role you play in offering it to yourself. **Provision is the resource of an intentional, optimal manner of offering ourselves available nourishment**. Although what we eat is certainly important and part of a lifestyle of mental wellness, the greater resource of provision is in the how, the ways we approach and consume food.

Approaching Provision When Food has been Problematic

Food is not an innocuous topic for many. A history of scarcity, starvation, or neglect can make a relationship with food painful and hold psychological distress in the long term (Myers, 2020). For those with disordered eating to any degree, the idea of focusing on food can feel problematic. As we've established with other resources, it's okay to begin with what's available to you. Approach this chapter cautiously if you need to. Begin at the margins of what and how you eat, places that feel accessible. We call this "working the edges," or approaching a problem at the shallows first. A useful quality of the resources is that you can choose when and how much you draw from them. They are available to you when you are ready to use them. Avoid forfeiting the entire resource because of limitations or obstacles. Draw what you can. Victory is often won by a narrow margin.

Perception of Food Matters

From how we think about food and how we select it, to what mindset we have when eating and how we actually eat our food, there are ways to optimize the process. There is fascinating research that points to the power our perception of food has on our actual digestion. The words used to describe food alters how we metabolize it. One such study used a smoothie-type beverage, bottled and packaged with two different labels. One label called the drink an "indulgence," while the other was "guilt free." Study participants drank the smoothie and then had their physiological responses measured. The result was a notable difference. Participants who "indulged" showed indicators of body chemistry more likely to gain weight and fat; participants who partook "guilt free" showed indicators of body chemistry less likely to gain weight, yet still felt hungry (Crum et al., 2011). A change in labeling changed the body's response.

Our bodies will draw more nutrients when we view the food as nutritious. We will gain less beneficial results and have lingering hunger when we consider a certain food as restrictive or unhealthy. We will feel more satiated when it is suggested we will. These suggestions regarding food are called "appetitive placebo effects," and they cause a change within the ventromedial prefrontal cortex (vmPFC) that can impact decision-making related to food and value assessment of how certain food aligns with our goals (Khalid et al., 2024). Beliefs about food have neurological implications that impact not only our relationship to food, but how our body responds to it. The mindset and language you use about the food in front of you can either maximize its benefit and gratification, or it can suppress the optimal value it could present to your system and mental health.

Consider the ways you present food to yourself and others. You may describe foods as healthy or unhealthy, good or bad. Perception can be influenced by thoughts, so the thoughts we choose to have about food matters. Appetizing. Threatening. Comforting. Essential. It could be any of these and more. Make no mistake, it will impact what your body will glean from the food you feed it. The way in which we market nourishment to ourselves will alter how we select it, how we digest it, how we metabolize it, and how it sustains us.

Viewing Food as Fuel for Life

For all that food can be, a neutral yet decidedly beneficial starting point is this: food is fuel. Love it or hate it, in plenty or in paltry, in delight or in disgust, food is what fuels us. It's fuel for the brain and body. It's fuel for the senses. It's fuel for connection as humans gather around it. Each of these facets of food as fuel have the capacity to impact mental wellness. In calling it fuel, we market it to ourselves as essential, useful, and rewarding, so our bodies are primed to receive it as such.

Viewing food as fuel is more potent when we connect it to the parts of life that matter most. I only put gas in my car because I have places to go. My various destinations make the fuel matter. Food serves a higher purpose when we connect it to the values and desired direction in our lives. If food is a distraction from our lives or if it's viewed as a threat to our desirability or well-being, the relationship will be more adversarial than it needs to be. To have a life-giving, positive relationship with food, our perspective may need to be more pragmatic. All that you must do and all that you love to do is powered by food. Food is not just calories or nutrients. It is fuel to live, and to live the purpose and fulfillment specific to you. Shifting your perspective to see food as the fuel for the best and most important things in your life will begin to shape the neurological and biological use of provision.

THE SCIENCE OF PROVISION

Provision is the resource of nourishment made more by the way we partake. **Provision provides ways to improve functioning of the brain and body by**

making what we eat and how we eat powerful partners for mental health. It's in the synergistic effect of food with mindset and technique. Our aim is not perfect execution with the best there is to get. It is gathering what is available to you, and using what is within your control to grow and sustain mental wellness.

Bio-Individuality and a Mindful Approach to Food

Bio-individuality is the idea that because humans are unique, approaches to health, including diet, cannot be one-size-fits-all. There's a reason why a health approach that worked for someone you know doesn't seem to work for you. You may not be doing it wrong, you're just not the same physical human being. Fingerprint, gut microbiome, hormones, genetics, and the rest all make you a different system. Therefore, it is necessary to "consider highly individualized characteristics" when it comes to nutrition (Lofft, 2020).

An emphasis on narrow nutrition advice for mental health gets tricky, because not only could it miss the bio-individual needs of a person but it can detract from the skill of attunement that clarifies the dietary needs for each individual. Therefore, I am not going to identify any specific diet here. Instead, the invitation stands to grow in awareness of your unique background, experience, and needs, and to respond to that awareness. "Nutritional conformity" may not serve a given individual's needs, disrupting health goals (Sedley, 2020). There are some specifics that you can apply with what you find does work for you. Begin gently shifting your attention from what works for others as a barometer of how you should eat, and give more attention to how your brain and body react to what and how you are eating.

There are resources, like water and food, that although every human has an intrinsic right to, access remains limited. Depending on context, access to food that research tells us is better for mental health is harder to come by for some (Crowe et al., 2018). So, although there may be specific foods claimed to improve depression, or about supplements purportedly likely to give you focus, or about diets heralded to decrease anxiety, you will not find any of that in this chapter. To stay on the target of resources that are available to every human, there needs to be a more inclusive lens that won't leave out large demographics due to access, culture, economics, and so forth. So, with the value of access and the reality of bio-individuality, the discussion of what to eat for mental health will be broad, adaptive, and focused on available essentials.

What We Eat Matters

Food and the way we eat it is one of the most in-your-control reservoirs available for your mental health. For our discussion, the word "diet" is not about what we restrict or how narrowly we keep our food intake tethered to specific goals. Our diet is simply the food we eat regularly, the fuel that serves our life at large. So, along with some considerations about what to eat, the greater idea is cultivating an approach to food that utilizes the brain-body connection effectively.

As we consider some of the foods that may improve your mental health, refrain from viewing each separate nutrient as a quid pro quo for a result.

> No univocal dietary component should be considered as a determinant for the improvement in mental health outcomes, while a general group of features of the whole dietary and eating habits seems to better describe the potential beneficial effects of diet with a synergistic interaction between different nutrients in the prevention of mental health disorders (Godos et al., 2020).

The real leverage seems to be in the overall force of what you eat in its entirety rather than a zero-sum game of good weighing out the bad. There are some general principles of what to eat for mental health that are worth noting, that you can apply to your way of eating at large, here and now.

"Food is some of the most potent mental health medicine available, with dietary interventions sometimes achieving similar results to specifically engineered pharmaceuticals, at a fraction of the price and with few if any side effects" (Naidoo, 2020). The specifics below are offered as a smorgasbord of options to either begin or deepen a familiarity with what food could have such powerful effects. Small, definite changes made incrementally are sufficient.

FATS AND PROTEIN

Painting with a broad brushstroke, there are some general concepts of what nourishment really alters mental wellness for the better. For starters, polyunsaturated fatty acids (PUFA), specifically Omega-3, have demonstrated support for the modulation of serotonin and dopamine (Godos et al., 2020). These real fats, or "healthy fats" as they are sometimes called, are necessary for baseline healthy brain functioning and can also intervene in disruptive symptoms of depression, ADHD, and even psychosis. For example, studies have shown that depression treatments rich in specific Omega-3 fatty acids outperform some pharmaceutical antidepressants

(Bentsen, 2017). Instead of processed seed oils or butter substitutes, consider if your mental health would be served by a diet rich in more real fats: olive oil, coconut oil, avocado, fish, organs, meat, nuts, and real butter.

Increasingly, psychologists are celebrating the role protein can play in stabilizing mental health by improving cognitive functioning as a whole (Dickerson et al., 2020), particularly when consumed early in the day. Proteins and amino acids play a role in quality of sleep, stress alleviation, and addressing fatigue (Godos et al., 2020). There are varying perspectives of which forms of protein are most advantageous for mental health. Furthermore, there are a variety of cultural or personal convictions that restrict consumption of certain proteins. The gist of it is to increase protein, earlier in the day, and in the simplest, least processed form you can.

Real fats and proteins are good starting points when we consider improving diet to improve mental health. Avoid starting by taking things away. Often, when people are looking to improve mental health, there is some form of mental duress present. Change can be hard, and beginning with deprivation or restriction can be damaging (Polivy, 1996). Better to begin by calling in the reinforcements of fat and protein.

Probiotics and the Microbiome

Besides providing nutrients, the food we consume can improve the body's ability to make use of the fuel we feed it. What we eat impacts the state of our microbiome, a powerhouse for all of wellness, including mental wellness. The microbiome (sometimes called the microbiota when speaking of specifics within the microbiome) is a habitat of microorganisms that, for our discussion, live within our gut (Berding et al., 2021). Turns out this habitat impacts not just digestion, but mental wellness as well. The microbiome is an integral part of neurological functioning.

It's like the various necessary parts of an online retailer. There are the "brains" of the operation, which would include those who work in the executive offices, coming up with the business plans and the prototypes of the products. The "brains" do not function in isolation. The vast, elaborate network of suppliers, distributors, and deliverers are an essential extension, working the exchange of goods in real time. Your brain may be the executive offices, hosting the brainstorming and the planning, but the functioning of your brain goes beyond its confines. The winding, unraveling network of nerves weaving throughout the body and even in your gut are the company's extension: suppliers, distributors, and deliverers of neurotransmitters.

Take serotonin, a vital neurotransmitter for mental wellness, most commonly associated with depressive symptoms because of its regulatory function. Ninety percent of serotonin receptors are actually found in the gut (Naidoo, 2020). The state of our microbiome directly influences serotonin and the mood it helps regulate (Brown and Liu, 2021), and that's just one example of "mental" action rooted in the gut. Depression and other "mental illnesses" are not confined to the wiring within the skull. It goes down through the stomach and into our intestines. Thankfully, the resource of provision is the most direct way to positively nurture this microbiome.

"The microbiota has emerged as a key player in regulating brain processes and behavior, via bidirectional communication" (Berding et al., 2021). Again, like an online supplier, the orders and products are not one-way messages. Returns and exchanges, suggested items, order information, and payment details are all relaying back and forth constantly. Similarly, the brain and gut are in constant communication, of which the microbiome is an integral component. "The bidirectional communication between the gut microbiota and the brain has been shown to influence neurotransmission and the behavior that is often associated with neuropsychiatric conditions" (Owen and Corfe, 2017). Just as our mindset and approach to providing ourselves with food impacts our processing of those nutrients, the habitat of our stomachs and intestines may or may not be in a state to best receive the food we are eating. Diet, or what we eat regularly, is a key factor in building up a thriving gut microbiota; and, like it or not, diet is increasingly identified as a significant player in optimal mental health (Berding et al., 2021).

Though many reach for supplemental versions of probiotics, I want to focus on food. Supplements are not accessible to everyone, and building up a healthy microbiome is feasible through what we eat, potentially more effectively through food than supplementation (Aslam et al., 2020). Eating probiotic foods is vital to mental health. Not only does it impact the environment of the gut, it also impacts the processing of other foods and the effectiveness they will have in supporting our mental health (Godos et al., 2020). Food that is not properly digested is not proper fuel.

Studies show a correlation with health of the gut microbiota and depressive symptoms and a responsivity to stress. There is "evidence for the potential of probiotics to improve anxiety, depression, and subjective stress in human populations" (Berding et al., 2021). Throughout human history, cultures around the world have had their unique versions of probiotic or fermented foods and beverages (Cuamatzin-Garcia et al., 2022). From yogurts and kefirs, kombucha and miso, sourdough bread and sauerkraut, probiotic foods have always been integral to human well-being (Aslam et al., 2020), and humans through the ages have worked to keep them nearby. Whichever probiotic food you find most accessible to you, eat it mindfully, and improve your mental well-being through that bidirectional communication pathway.

Eat Real Food

Humans, who are inherently omnivores, "consume a combination of food groups with every meal and studying single foods could overlook the potential synergistic effect dietary compliments might have" (Berding et al., 2021). Hence, a realistic focus on a diet for the average person to improve their mental health should focus more on the big picture, rather than a grocery list of "shoulds" and "shouldn'ts."

Studies consistently show that "the more one eats a highly processed diet, the more one is at risk for developing psychiatric symptoms, such as depression and anxiety" (Owen and Corfe, 2017). Avoiding processed foods does not mean more expensive food, but it usually means simpler food. Real food, that is food that is less processed, is going to typically have more nutrients that will translate to more bioavailable fuel for your life.

In my clinical observation, there are two main obstacles to people eating enough real food for their mental health. First, some aren't eating enough, often accompanied by a noticeable health- or image-consciousness, and so they aren't getting or able to maintain necessary fuel by unnecessary restriction (Genton et al., 2015). Second, some are eating large quantities of food but are still malnourished for the lack of real food in their diet (Sukol, 2019). The imbalance may come from an unfamiliarity with bio-individuality and a disconnection from how food affects well-being. It also may come from misinformation. In studies done on health misinformation, inaccurate information reached almost 90% of consumers, and specifically, over a third of diet and nutrition related content was misinformation (Suarez-Lledo & Alvarez-Galvez, 2021). Whether due to misinformation or the nuances that come with bio-individuality, people are often eating in a way that they believe is right for them, but in actuality is resulting in a deficit of real food. In either scenario, the answer is the same: eat enough actual real food for your brain and body.

How We Eat Matters

The most important aspect of provision for mental health is what is within your control. Perhaps part of that is what you eat, the actual foods and nutrients you consume. More certain than that, you have more control over how you eat. Mindset and demeanor, from expressions of gratitude to how slow you chew, the act of feeding yourself can be done in a way to directly provide mental health support. The idea of eating differently may seem unremarkable, and so the change anticipated appears trivial. With the weight of mental health burdens and the ubiquitous presence of food in daily living, small changes produce profound improvements (Owen and Corfe, 2017). The changes may include what we eat, but it must certainly include how we eat.

Eat Fuel

Perception is foundational in the work of changing how we eat for mental wellness. In saying we should "eat fuel," the emphasis is on mindset in how we relate to food. Taking from the previously mentioned research, the way a food product is marketed and the way we view it changes how our body biologically processes it. The same food consumed with different mindsets produces different results (Khalid et al., 2024).

Too often, people maintain narratives about food from a deficiency standpoint, and these perspectives of food will impact health (Bickel et al., 2017). We may view it as "not enough," "unhealthy," or "unpalatable." Though these descriptors may hold some truth, if they are the primary descriptors used when we approach food, our entire brain-body system is primed to receive that food through that filter. Terms of "not enough" may leave us feeling unsatisfied. Terms of "unhealthy" may result in physiologically forfeiting some of the nutrients available while also leaving emotional guilt or concern about connected health problems. Contrariwise, viewing food as fuel benefits the systems. Though the food in front of you may not be sufficient, wholesome, or delicious, it is still needed, beneficial fuel. By calling it as such, our brains and bodies are then prepared to take in the most benefit possible.

A narrative of food as fuel, conjures a mindset of expectancy, appreciation, and energy. These are beneficial to the brain-body system trying to make the most of what we're eating. When we are in a state of appreciation, the nervous system is regulated (McCraty & Childre, 2004), which allows for the body to be in a proper state for digestion and other crucial functions that only happen with the parasympathetic nervous system (Tindle & Tadi, 2022). Beyond "fuel," we are free to explore additional language that can mechanistically optimize the way we provide food to ourselves in alignment with our values and goals.

Eat Slow

We've already discussed how the way we view food changes how we digest and process it. The health of our digestion impacts the nutrients going to our brain. Eating slow while engaging the senses leads to better digestion and use of nourishment. Taking our time to eat slowly not only allows us time to chew properly for optimal absorption of nutrients but also encourages use of all the senses for increased pleasure, reducing physiological symptoms of stress (Lyzwinski et al., 2019). Eating slowly uses our exteroceptive senses of sight, smell, taste, and so forth, as well as calling upon interoceptive awareness to aid in connection to our appetite, hunger, and feelings of satisfaction. There's a double benefit to it: not only are we eating more functionally from a nutrition standpoint, but we are also supporting the brain-body partnership. Awareness, senses, and the slowing of the breath that are necessary in eating slower provide desirable neurological benefits.

Food is not just for fuel of the brain and body, though that is a primary function. It also is fuel for the senses, for enjoyment. Eating for pleasure is often seen in a villainous light, as if it only serves as a culprit of unwanted weight gain and health disruption. However, in the right mindset, eating for pleasure can enhance well-being. The key, once again, is in how we eat for pleasure. A healthy relationship with food is gained by using the senses, slowing down to tune in to the whole body experience of eating, and by being mindful of past enjoyable experiences associated with a particular food (Bédard et al., 2020). If there are certain ways of eating that align with our values and our goals, we can cultivate these dietary patterns through pleasure and slowing down with the senses.

As we noted with the power of marketing, how we present our regular, daily food to ourselves can make even the simplest of meals rich with holistic satisfaction. A slice of freshly baked bread with a thick layer of butter. An apple, perfectly cool, crisp, and fragrant. Fluffy, warm rice with a dusting of salt and pepper. Deep breaths, all senses stirred, one uninterrupted minute devoted to eating, and the mind can make the most of basic sustenance, for the body and the brain.

Eat with People, Sometimes

Sharing the table can be heartening, and we should seek out opportunities to eat meals with others. Those who regularly eat socially or with loved ones have better life satisfaction, experience more trust in their relationships, and are in a better mood overall. It is also interesting to note that shared eating preceded improved relationships, and not the valued relationship improving the experience of food (Dunbar, 2017). Indeed, food is fuel for relationships.

And yet, it goes both ways. We may think that our food choices are largely a product of will. As if a specific calculation of what is best will ultimately determine what choice I should make. Humans aren't that robotic. We are shaped by the people around us in making food choices. "Whom you eat with is more powerful than nature in determining food habits" (Wilson, 2015). Not only is food a fuel for our relationships, but our relationships shape our experience of provision.

It must also be noted that eating with others can have its pitfalls. Eating while in sympathetic nervous system dominance, that state of alarm and disruption, hinders digestion as well as the variety of benefits that come with eating (Cherpak, 2019). There are some contexts when eating with others is decidedly trying. Indeed, there are many reasons that mealtimes could be difficult: being a parent or caregiver responsible for feeding another person, meals with those with whom you may have conflict, or eating at home when that is not a safe place to be. Pursue peaceful times to eat with others, and eat alone when you need to. And at all times, eat slowly and savor the fuel available to you.

PROVISION IN PRACTICE

Food is fuel for the brain and body, as well as fuel for the senses, fuel for gathering with others, and fuel for the most meaningful parts of life. By making small, piecemeal changes to what we eat and how we eat, we supply ourselves with more robust mental wellness. Remember again that due to bio-individuality, the fuel that is "better" for someone else may not be the same for you. **We practice provision by incremental alterations of what, how, and why we eat in everyday practice for everyday change**.

Meditation Practice – A Guided Practice for Brain-Body Communication in Provision

Interoception and sensory engagement assist in forming neural connections that posture the brain and body for an improved, mindful relationship with food. The emphasis is on a receptive mindset that welcomes the fuel available from nutrition to sensation. Go to kristaagler.com/book/keepinmind to listen to the provided audio or follow the accompanying prompts for a guided meditation on a brain-body connection with provision.

Table 9.1 *Cultivating a Provision Mindset*

Prompt	Response
Identify activities you enjoy that require energy.	
Identify some ways food helps your body.	
Identify positive experiences connected to the smell or taste of specific foods. Note them.	
Identify eating traditions you value.	
Complete the sentences below using the responses above.	
Food allows me to: ______________________________	
Food serves my body by: ______________________________	
When I taste or smell ________________, I remember: ________________	
Food is a meaningful, important part of my life, particularly with______________________________.	

Reflection Practice – Cultivating a Provision Mindset

Like any mindset, we develop a kind and helpful way of thinking about food through practice. With some of your identified values and desired life direction in mind, complete Table 9.1 to clarify an adaptive mindset regarding food. For one week, it may be helpful to read the completed sentences from this practice each day. Observe any shifts in mindset or relationship to food from the practice.

***Table 9.2** Mindful Alterations to Fuel*

Type of fuel: protein, fat, or probiotic	*Form of that fuel: (meat, yogurt, etc)*	*Time of day consumed:*	*Immediate observations or mindful appreciation:*	*End of day observations of overall effects:*

Conscious Practice – Mindful Alterations to Fuel

Read through the potential additions listed in Table 9.2 to fuel your mental wellness. Consider starting with one. If you feel so inclined, add as many as you'd like. If you're not sure where to begin, try this: probiotic food daily, protein in the mornings, fats at each meal. Notice how your body responds. Perhaps including these foods in your regular diet is already the norm for you. Use the following practice as an opportunity to strengthen the mental connection between those foods and direct impact on your mental health. Visualize with appreciation the fuel that these specific foods provide.

Remember bio-individuality and honor the uniqueness of your system. What works for someone else may not work for you. Pay attention to indicators that a certain way of eating is working for you: energy, digestion, mental clarity, and so on. Furthermore, if you have any medical conditions or are under the treatment of a physician, include them in decision-making of any major dietary changes.

Lifestyle Practice – Partake of Daily Provision with Intention

Cultivate awareness of the things you do, without judgment, to feed yourself. Notice your speed, intentionality, choice, distraction, enjoyment, frustration, autopilot. Whatever your experience with eating, notice it. Acknowledge the act of feeding yourself. If you rely on others to eat, acknowledge that connection with similar observations. Then draw attention to connect the act of eating with your daily functioning. The activities that make up your daily life, enjoyable or hard, meaningful or mundane, necessary or for pleasure, are all fueled by the food you offer yourself, and the way you do so. Keep in mind what specific activities food fuels in your life.

IN SUMMARY

There are essential nutrients that benefit mental health, and yet, beyond what we eat, how we eat is a factor within our control to capitalize on our food intake and pursue mental wellness. We can do so by practicing the following: Eat for fuel. Eat real. Eat slow. Eat with others. Fuel your brain and body. Fuel your senses. Fuel your relationships. Fuel what matters most to you with provision.

With food, what may be readily available to some is scarce to others. In places and situations where food and water are scarce, there are other menacing factors creating increased rates of anxiety, depression, and trauma. Perhaps part of your practice of provision is contributing to making food accessible to those who need it. Begin with those closest to you, offering food to people you see regularly. Then consider local food pantries, organizations, or ministries that provide food for your community. Perhaps also consider national or global movements to address food crises.

Perhaps we will gain even more from provision as we make it available to others. Feeding others fills us. As we are influenced by the people with whom we share tables, we influence others by making nourishment available in more ways than just providing calories. When we offer fuel to others, we improve the table, and the mental health landscape, for all of us.

REFERENCES

Aslam, H., Green, J., Jacka, F. N., Collier, F., Berk, M., Pasco, J., & Dawson, S. L. (2020). Fermented foods, the gut and mental health: a mechanistic overview with implications for depression and anxiety. *Nutritional Neuroscience, 23*(9), 659–671.

Bédard, A., Lamarche, P. O., Grégoire, L. M., Trudel-Guy, C., Provencher, V., Desroches, S., & Lemieux, S. (2020). Can eating pleasure be a lever for healthy eating? A systematic scoping review of eating pleasure and its links with dietary behaviors and health. *PloS One, 15*(12), Article e0244292.

Bentsen, H. (2017). Dietary polyunsaturated fatty acids, brain function and mental health. *Microbial Ecology in Health and Disease, 28*(sup1), Article 1281916.

Berding, K., Vlckova, K., Marx, W., Schellekens, H., Stanton, C., Clarke, G., Jacka, F., Dinan, T. G., & Cryan, J. F. (2021). Diet and the microbiota–gut–brain axis: sowing the seeds of good mental health. *Advances in Nutrition, 12*(4), 1239–1285.

Bickel, W. K., Stein, J. S., Moody, L. N., Snider, S. E., Mellis, A. M., & Quisenberry, A. J. (2017). Toward narrative theory: Interventions for reinforcer pathology in health behavior. *Impulsivity: How Time and Risk Influence Decision Making,* 227–267.

Brown, A., & Liu, H. (2021). Interaction between intestinal serotonin and the gut microbiome. *International Journal of Anatomy and Physiology,* 7(04), 192–196.

Cherpak, C. E. (2019). Mindful eating: a review of how the stress-digestion-mindfulness triad may modulate and improve gastrointestinal and digestive function. *Integrative Medicine: A Clinician's Journal, 18*(4), 48.

Crowe, J., Lacy, C., & Columbus, Y. (2018). Barriers to food security and community stress in an urban food desert. *Urban Science, 2*(2), 46–46.

Crum, A. J., Corbin, W. R., Brownell, K. D., & Salovey, P. (2011). Mind over milkshakes: mindsets, not just nutrients, determine ghrelin response. *Health Psychology: Official Journal of the Division of Health Psychology, American Psychological Association, 30*(4), 424–9.

Cuamatzin-García, L., Rodríguez-Rugarcía, P., El-Kassis, E. G., Galicia, G., Meza-Jiménez, M. de L., Baños-Lara, M. D. R., Zaragoza-Maldonado, D. S., & Pérez-Armendáriz, B. (2022). Traditional fermented foods and beverages from around the world and their health benefits. *Microorganisms, 10*(6).

Dickerson, F., Gennusa, J. V., 3rd, Stallings, C., Origoni, A., Katsafanas, E., Sweeney, K., Campbell, W. W., & Yolken, R. (2020). Protein intake is associated with cognitive functioning in individuals with psychiatric disorders. *Psychiatry Research, 284,* Article 112700.

Dunbar, R. I. (2017). Breaking bread: the functions of social eating. *Adaptive Human Behavior and Physiology, 3*(3), 198–211.

Genton, L., Cani, P. D., & Schrenzel, J. (2015). Alterations of gut barrier and gut microbiota in food restriction, food deprivation and protein-energy wasting. *Clinical Nutrition, 34*(3), 341–349.

Godos, J., Currenti, W., Angelino, D., Mena, P., Castellano, S., Caraci, F., Galvano, F., Del Rio, D., Ferri, R., & Grosso, G. (2020). Diet and mental health: review of the recent updates on molecular mechanisms. *Antioxidants (Basel), 9*(4).

Khalid, I., Rodrigues, B., Dreyfus, H., Frileux, S., Meissner, K., Fossati, P., Hare, T. A., & Schmidt, L. (2024). Mapping expectancy-based appetitive placebo effects onto the brain in women. *Nature Communications, 15*(1), 248.

Lofft, Z. (2020). When social media met nutrition: How influencers spread misinformation, and why we believe them. *Health Science Inquiry, 11*(1), 56–61.

Lyzwinski, L. N., Edirippulige, S., Caffery, L., & Bambling, M. (2019). Mindful eating mobile health apps: review and appraisal. *Jmir Mental Health, 6*(8), Article 12820.

McCraty, R., & Childre, D. (2004). Chapter 12 - The Grateful Heart The Psychophysiology of Appreciation. *The Psychology of Gratitude, 230.*

Myers, C. A. (2020). Food insecurity and psychological distress: A review of the recent literature. *Current nutrition reports, 9*(2), 107–118.

Naidoo, U. (2020). *This is your brain on food: An indispensable guide to the surprising foods that fight depression, anxiety, PTSD, OCD, ADHD, and more.* Little, Brown Spark.

Owen, L., & Corfe, B. (2017). The role of diet and nutrition on mental health and well-being. *Proceedings of the Nutrition Society, 76,* 425–426.

Polivy, J. (1996). Psychological consequences of food restriction. *Journal of the American Dietetic Association, 96*(6), 589–592.

Sedley, L. (2020). Advances in nutritional epigenetics—A fresh perspective for an old idea. Lessons learned, limitations, and future directions. *Epigenetics Insights, 13.*

Suarez-Lledo, V., & Alvarez-Galvez, J. (2021). Prevalence of health misinformation on social media: systematic review. *Journal of Medical Internet Research, 23*(1), Article e17187.

Sukol, R. B. (2019). Obesity: A Malnourished State—Real Food Is the Answer. *Alternative and Complementary Therapies, 25*(5), 234–237.

Tindle, J., & Tadi, P. (2022). Neuroanatomy, parasympathetic nervous system. StatPearls Publishing.

Wilson, B. (2015). *First bite: How we learn to eat.* Basic Books.

Chapter 10

Rhythm: A Resource of Biology, Rest, and Predictability

The last few years had been unexpectedly eventful for Sam. At fifty-eight years old, he thought life would settle down. Established high up in his company, he was successful in business. He was good at it. He had started working at sixteen, after his father left his mom and three younger siblings. He took care of his family until all his siblings were grown and his mom was stable. He met a woman, got married, and started working at the company he's been with ever since. They had two kids, both adolescents, when the pandemic hit.

His wife had loved her job waiting tables at an upscale restaurant, but being at home and unable to contribute instigated a troubling battle with depression. Their son, who had always struggled academically, fell significantly behind with the changes at his school. All this, Sam would say, they could have figured out. But then their daughter was diagnosed with an aggressive form of cancer, and their entire life changed. Jobs were put on the back burner, school was an afterthought, and they reoriented their lives to treatment, traveling to and from appointments and hospital stays. Eventually, surprisingly and thankfully, she recovered.

Sam and his family worked hard to right the ship, and they did. Part of that work for him was going to therapy to address the traumatic reactions his brain and body had to watching his daughter's illness and reckoning with the real possibility of her death. He completed trauma treatment and maintained therapy on a monthly basis "just because." A couple years after his daughter went into remission, he anticipated stopping therapy for good, but just as the winter turned into spring, Sam began to struggle unexpectedly. His anxiety returned, full tilt, and he felt on edge most of the time. He also described a constant ache and pressure on his chest.

DOI: 10.4324/9781003521945-13

Discouraged, he talked to his therapist about what could be responsible for this sudden change when he had been doing so well. They discussed his lifestyle, looking for any changes to diet, routine, work stress, or other potential factors. In resignation, Sam tossed his hands up and expressed that he always had a hard time in the spring, at least for the last six years. When asked about any significance spring might have for him in recent years, he reflected. He shook his head no, and paused, continuing to think back. "Well, my mom died in April eight years ago. We knew it was coming, and it was as peaceful as could be expected. You think that could be it?"

For Sam, grief was held in pattern with the seasons, hibernating most of the year and then pushing to the surface. Since his mom's death, the pervasive sadness was difficult to address as he also felt relief when the years of being responsible for her came to an end. The guilt kept him from grief. His biological clock, now connected to loss, reminded him year after year, until he could "take care of the real business." Wisdom from walking through his daughter's cancer allowed him to respond to the clock and grieve effectively for the first time.

THE NATURE OF RHYTHM

Along with all living creatures, the natural order of humanity necessitates alignment with certain rhythms. The course of life is set by the things we do regularly. There are some habits we've come by naturally or that come easy to us. There are others we have built into our lives either by design, desire, or necessity. There are patterns of action, thought, speaking, location, proximity, exposure, consumption, and expending, among others. Additionally, there are internal clocks that function as built-in rhythms that we can work with or against. How we steward each of our patterns directly contributes to our mental state.

The chapter on span displayed the importance of limits to maximize capacity. In a similar yet distinct way, rhythm sets pace and stride for daily living in a way that positively impacts mental health. Whereas span is about limits, like an out-of-bounds line, rhythm is more about pace, as in a time-out. Span is spatial. Rhythm is tempo.

Rhythm, Patterns for Mental Health

Rhythm is a regular, repeated pattern. When it comes to mental health, rhythm refers to patterns of living that can reliably move us toward mental wellness. In music, an established rhythm can carry a song. It forms the scaffolding around which the melodious and the lyrical can take shape. Similarly, the life rhythm we construct becomes a characterizing, driving force to bring us along in a given direction. The influence rhythm has in its repetition and expressive nature means it has the potential to improve or impair.

There are specific aspects of the brain and body that work in tandem with aspects of our outer environment and our internal systems (Schulz, 2007). Like tides and constellations, the human mind is patterned and seems meant to follow certain courses. To fall out of these rhythms is to run the risk of disrupting mental health. Indeed, practically all mental illness diagnoses correlate to disruptions of these biological rhythms (Foster & Kreitzman, 2014). In addition to the biological mechanisms of rhythm, psychologically there are benefits to finding rhythms of habit in mindful balance (Fujiwara et al., 2022).

Rhythm is a resource of pacing and priority that tunes our patterns to benefit mental wellness. Rhythm encourages certain elements of autopilot to be beneficial. It reduces the energy required for practices that, once established, bring continued advantage for our mental well-being. Not everything should be on autopilot or left to habit; however, recreating the wheel each day drains valuable energy. Rhythm primes some of our helpful operations to become standard, propelling us forward. It optimizes both daily habits as well as needed new practices as they become reliable, gaining momentum toward mental wellness.

Bio-Individuality of Rhythms

Rhythm, as a mental health resource, is fluid. With bio-individuality at play, it will be unique to each person, but some principles are true to us all (Schulz, 2007). Understanding the resource will focus on those common characteristics that make up the human rhythm. The ever important skill of interoception will be needed to take the general concepts of the natural human rhythms to be effectively applied to your specific biology, psychology, season, and way of living.

I see bio-individuality most clearly when I consider my kids' patterns in juxtaposition with my own. When they sleep and for how long, and especially when they wake up, stands in stark contrast to my internal tendency. The frequency with which they seek out snacks and the timing of their bursts of energy seem often contradictory to what seems natural to me. There are biological mechanisms at play that change throughout the lifespan responsible for the differences (Olejniczak et al., 2023). Indeed, there are differences biologically from person-to-person. Therefore, we would do well to be conscious of how we set our rhythms, not keeping time merely by those around us or even by general consensus. Optimal use of this resource requires a mindful responsiveness in the feedback loop between our internal responses and the environment around us.

THE SCIENCE OF RHYTHM

In exploring rhythm and how it serves mental wellness, we will look at three important patterns: rhythms of biology, rhythms of rest, and rhythms of predictability. Understanding our internal clocks, human behavioral components, and environmental factors will help shape better rhythms.

Rhythm provides internal and external regulation, cultivating consistency and momentum in mental wellness. Our brains need action and stillness, go and pause, light and dark, work and rest. They need them at specific times and in specific ways (Schulz, 2007). When we identify and acknowledge the patterns best suited for our brains and bodies, an internal pacing is born in which mental functioning becomes more like renewable energy, recharging before hitting empty. Mental health then shifts from a sense of a constant uphill trudge to one of propelled, sustainable movement.

Rhythms of Biology

It has long been understood that nature is patterned and rhythmic. Chronobiology is the study of those rhythms of a biological nature with three components: happening recurrently, organized in some measure of time, and impacting physiology (Moreno et al., 2019). Against our nature, we may orient and pace in step with the technological world, rather than the biological one to which we belong. Sometimes called "body rhythms," there are repeating ebbs and flows at the molecular level, impacting and shaped by hormones, environment, psychology, among others (Bilal & Naveed, 2022). Humans experience such ordering along with the opening and closing morning glory, the migration patterns of the swallows of Capistrano, and the nightly activity and daily sleep patterns of bats (Zhang, et al., 2022). Plants and animals alike follow biological rhythms, and not just one simple clock per species. Within a single organism, different organs and neural connections follow their own "clocks" programmed down into cells all throughout the body (Moreno et al., 2019). There is a deep, calculated organization responsible for the flourishing of all organic life. The same is true of you. You don't simply have a "biological clock" or a broad brushstroke of a "circadian rhythm"; you are fashioned to function according to a number of clocks throughout the different systems of your body, like differently sized cogs keeping independent time to run the machine that is you. Machine is not quite the right word. You're far more complex, intuitive, and alive.

Circadian and Other Biological Clocks

By far, the circadian rhythm is the body clock most commonly known. In part that's for good reason because the impact to our day-to-day life is perhaps most observable with the circadian clock. It is important, but it's not the only one. Briefly, I want to touch on some of the others, to begin to paint the picture of how very metrical we are.

Biological clocks have long been observed. The circadian clock represents a period of approximately, not exactly, 24 hours. Circaseptan rhythms recur every seven days, with the circalunar repeating in time with the moon (Raible et al., 2017). We, along with a lot of nature, function on some circannual or seasonal clocks, repeating on the yearly (Pengelley, 2012). Not all clocks fall so neatly in step with our concepts of time. Our body also has what is called ultradian rhythms, which represents those biological patterns that cycle in under 24 hours. Complementary to that, the infradian rhythms are those that are longer than 24 hours, but not up to the seven days of the circaseptan (Bilal & Naveed, 2022). If you think of each varietal of biological clock like its own piece of a drum kit, you start to get the sense that your systems function with jazzlike animation and depth. Neurotransmitters, hormones, digestion, breathing, muscle tone, blood vessel constriction, and appetites are just some of the clock-influenced systems at work.

It's all happening simultaneously, and the timing can get thrown off in one area, affecting the others. When people go to therapy to address mental disruption, it's not uncommon for there to be confusion about what is "off" or what is the root of the mental disruption. Understanding brings clarity, and so it is relevant to understand, even at a surface level, the various clocks at work in our functioning. It's possible you're not inexplicably "off" – you may be out of sync. It's possible you're not chronically fatigued – perhaps you are sleeping in irregular patterns. You may not be distractible and unproductive – you may have a system unsure of what's next and seeking to be active at suboptimal times. An appreciation of biological clocks and their effect is an essential in basic mental health.

Biological Clocks and Mental Health

The circadian rhythm, as the skeleton shaping our daily pace, is a good place to begin dialing in, correcting what has fallen out of time. "Circadian rhythms are recurring cycles that display periods of about twenty four hours, and are manifested across a range of behavioral, physiological, and cognitive processes" (Coogan, 2013). In other words, just about everything you do can either impact or be impacted by your circadian rhythm. Within that approximate 24-hour window, there is a time to sleep, times to eat, times to be productive, times to rest. There are times to exert energy and times for the brain and body to do important rebuilding work from muscles to body chemistry. There are times that are more optimal than others for each function.

The circadian and other body rhythms are integral in recovery from neuronal stress and initiate neuronal repair. They are involved in the regulation of many of our neurotransmitters, essential in balanced and optimal mental health functioning. Initial observations in research connecting the disruption of circadian rhythms with mood disorders began more than 60 years ago (Coogan, 2013). The concept is not new or really up for debate. The nature of the connection continues to be studied, and what we can do to counter the mood disruption is similarly a point of focus in the field. Mood shifts within episodes of depression follow the circadian variance. Circadian disruption can also be linked to anxiety, stress, and sleep disruption. It is linked at a general level to mental illness (Bilal & Naveed, 2022). It may be important to note that there is debate about whether disrupted circadian rhythm causes mental disruption, or if it's the other way around. The evidence from both sides seems to indicate that both have the capacity to influence the other. Either way, it may be important to remember that depression is not a traceable disease but a term used to describe a disorder characterized by a certain set of symptoms that can come from a number of different root causes. Suffice it to say, to struggle with low mood, significant sadness, sporadic anxiety, or other mental dysregulation is to necessitate a look at your daily rhythms.

Mechanisms of Biological Clocks

Body clocks are ultimately driven by genetics, though they follow a combination of internal and external cues (Panda, 2020). The study of plants, animals, and humans when it comes to chronobiology paints a fascinating picture of an unseen inward timekeeper. Plants, even in a room without windows, will raise and lower their leaves in time with their intended purpose of sun exposure. Our clocks are ticking with our genetic download, which means it's important to remember once again our bio-individuality. As genetics differ, there can be variance in optimal functioning of clocks. There are general specifics, but there is also nuance. Any study that shows how it works for a majority percentage still leaves a percentage for whom the studied outcome does not apply. Our aim is to continually pivot toward the aspects of each resource that are within our control. Parts of our biological clocks are beyond our influence, so we will focus on the parts that are impressionable.

Enter the external components in the regulation of our biological rhythms. They are referred to as zeitgebers, a word meaning "time cues" (Coogan, 2013). There are two zeitgebers that are largely responsible for external regulation and also are largely within our influence: light exposure and scheduling. We are not in search of hard rules. That would not be accessible to all, considering the significant lifestyle limitations and variance in biology to each person. Still, there are general concepts that can guide our awareness and the percussion of our daily living.

Through the light that hits the eyes (in the photoreceptive retinal ganglion cells), the circadian phase keeps tempo. Light is a way we can "entrain" our circadian clock, which is often thrown off by our unintended misuse of light (Coogan, 2013). You could read different sources and get specific time frames and set numbers of hours for sun exposure. I want to avoid doing that here, again for accessibilities sake. There are a few helpful generalizations.

First, as much as possible, sleep should line up with dark and being awake should line up with light (Foster & Kreitzman, 2014). Geography, work shift, health, responsibilities, and other factors may make that difficult, but it's a helpful general guideline. We're aiming for being awake with the light and sleeping when it's dark. Second, view light, preferably natural, as soon as is reasonable after waking. It's a strong, pacing zeitgeber for the circadian rhythm while also boasting antidepressant effects (Blume et al., 2019). Third, the pattern of each day should be principally repeatable. Think about if you have a late night. You stay up hours later than you usually do, and then perhaps you sleep in the next day hours later than you typically would. The number of hours of sleep was the same, but the subsequent fatigue is still staggering. It's a disruption of clock rather than a deficit of sleep, and the effect can last for days (Moreno et al., 2019).

Scheduling of sleep, activity, and eating also has significant influence on circadian rhythm, and the health of these dynamics is an output of the circadian rhythm as well as some of the other clocks at play (Moreno et al., 2019). It's a two-way route of communication within the body and within the brain-body connection. So beyond light and sleep, the regularity of when we do straining activities and when we eat is part of the percussion of all our systems. For those activities to be regularly unpredictable can lead to problems for some, perhaps for many. Again, I caution against strict response to these points. The goal is healthy and reliable regularity, not rigidity.

A Note on Circannual Rhythms

Circannual rhythms, or the biological clocks functioning on a yearly basis, "are controlled in part by exposure to earth's light-dark cycle resulting from the 23.5 degree tilt of the earth on its axis, its daily rotation, and the annual orbit around the sun, as well as from climatic weather patterns" (Moreno et al., 2019). Just like many animal species evolutionarily learn to expect different weather, food availability, and conditions for reproduction based on the seasons that make up a year, our brains and bodies follow similar patterns in response to seasonal zeitgebers as well as the internal genetic pace.

Mental health can be impacted by experience. There are mood, behavioral, and biological processes within our mental health driven by the circannual rhythm (Mutak & Vukasović Hlupić, 2017). These circannual rhythms come into play with memories related to loss or trauma, causing the body to prepare for what it biologically learned happened in certain times of the year. Due to the very wide lens that is a year, it may be difficult to see annual patterns in your biology and psychology, unless your life or work is tied to the calendar like teachers and farmers. Without consistent cues, the aspects of our mental and emotional well-being that are tied to the circannual rhythm may be difficult to detect, but it is something to consider, especially in moments where you sense your mental wellness is unexpectedly struggling.

Rhythms of Rest

Rhythm is about balancing the outputs with inputs. In poetry, there are rhythms formed by stressed and unstressed syllables. The poetics of living require both the stressed syllables of output tempered by the unstressed syllables of rest. Rest is not absence or shutting down; it is an intentional, rich complement to the taxation of that which requires work. Clinically, I have observed mental health distress in direct correlation with lack of rest. Too often, it seems people wait until they are past limits to consider taking a rest. It's viewed as a life preserve rather than as a regular, commonplace, household pillar in the day-to-day cadence. That's not rest; that's recovery.

Denying rest puts the brain in a state that struggles to accurately assess and meet needs (Asp, 2015). Regular intervals of rest help our brains assess when we are ready to work and when we need to pause. The more we nurture this skill, the more finely tuned it becomes. Regular rest also integrates predictability of when the next break is coming, reducing the drive to hoard times of nonwork. Regular rest strengthens the learned neural pathways associated with the parasympathetic nervous system, improving cognition, focus, satisfaction, creativity, among many others.

Rest is an action we take, and a state we occupy for a time. It is characterized as free from labor and pressure. It is purposeful restoration, enjoyable and receptive. It involves movement away from or distinct from that which is "nonrest" (Asp, 2015). It is the strengthening that comes with a decided pause.

There are two parts of the brain at play when it comes to rest. First there is the "resting-state functional connectivity," which is basically the brain's capacity to make use of rest, restoring energy and connections, while doing passive but necessary work that improves active work. Second, there is the default mode network (DMN), the part of the brain that is still active when we ourselves seem to not be (Kral et al., 2019). We each differ in our current capacity to access the resource of rest. Some have schedules, lifestyles, or cultural contexts more favorable to rest than others. There are ways intention and choice can bring change, even within those environments. Some have a better brain disposition to rest and make the most of it. This too is changeable by use and repeated use. Rest belongs as a rhythm rather than a lifeline. We get better at resting and letting rest make us better the more we do it. Through regular, repeated practices of rest, we can invest in optimizing both our "resting-state functional connectivity" and the DMN.

The Example of Sabbath-Keeping

Across cultures and throughout time, there are many practices of regular rest. "Sabbath-keeping" is one cultural and holistic example of a regular rhythm of rest named from the Hebrew word "sabat," meaning "to cease, desist, or put to an end" (Diddams et al., 2004). The ancient Hebrew practice of Sabbath is a weekly day of rest. From sunset Friday through sunset on Saturday, work is halted both professionally and in the home. Attention is given to slowing down, quality time with the family and the community, and spiritual observation. Boundaries are created between work and other arenas of life.

With some practices of Sabbath, "people find respite or experience less stress by inserting 'punctuation' around their activities each week" (Diddams et al., 2004). Though the practice is honored as a faith tradition, it taps into mental well-being, decreasing anxiety and depressive symptoms, improving self-control, and encouraging gratitude and life satisfaction (Proeschold-Bell et al., 2022). Such whole-life exhaling and subsequent enrichment is available to us in prioritizing pauses for rest on purpose and in a manner that can be anticipated. Rest being anticipated, knowing that it's coming, is important for the pacing of rest. Part of the pull of a good rhythm in music is that you can sing or dance along, anticipating the beat. So we come to the role of predictability.

Rhythms of Predictability

The unexpected in life, even if it is pleasant, has an activating effect on the brain. We likely have awareness of the experience with noticeable upsets or significant surprises, yet even the seemingly benign or imperceptible unexpected moments are experienced in our brain a certain way (Gu et al., 2020). Conversely, when events are expected, even boring, the brain and nervous system are more prone to more subdued states. Building in more predictability in purposeful and calculated spaces can have positive and calming benefits for our mental wellness.

When a behavior or practice becomes routine, it becomes a habit. Whether or not a habit is life-giving depends partially on the quality of the repetitive action. Not all patterns are created equal. A pattern or habit can also become problematic when it becomes inflexible, even if it's a "healthy" or "positive" one. If we look at rhythm like the speed of a car, its variability depending on the situation and setting is necessary for its usefulness. It is important to keep flexibility; routines or rules added to life unnecessarily, even when positive, can add a "should" perspective that is counterproductive to mental health, causing more strain than reprieve (Diddams et al., 2004). Mindful balance is key.

Routines are powerful tools for our mental health, because their effect is layered. Once established, the predictability itself provides a sense of calm and of rootedness (Fujiwara et al., 2022). They also can be created and shaped with practices that are themselves consistent with our values and desired direction. Again, think of percussion. The different styles of drum and changing the quality of the instrument will impact the sound that is produced. So the beat matters and the chosen instrument matters. The predictability of a rhythm matters; the quality of the activities you build it with also matters.

Uncertainty, the kind that negatively impacts mental stability, relates to whether something around us will happen, what the nature of that something is, and when that something will occur (Gu et al., 2020). Clearly, that can apply to a lot of things, and research indicates we experience the negative effects of uncertainty as relates to everyday life situations, not just catastrophizing worst-case scenarios. When we build routines that give some predictability to the whether and the what and the when of our daily lives, we are safeguarding against the negative effects of uncertainty, which cannot be totally eliminated. Nor should it be. We can't eliminate uncertainty; we can, with what's within our control, create degrees of predictability.

Predictability with exteroceptive stimuli is useful in bolstering mental health (Tan et al., 2019). The five senses of smell, sight, taste, sound, and touch can be intentionally manipulated with regularity. We can approach this a couple ways. Consider how some places you prefer to be have a level of sensory familiarity to them. Many of these associations between specific senses and certain positive states of mind happened passively over time. The opportunity is available to us to proactively create such associations and familiarity. Furthermore, we can also practice regular mindfulness, keeping our senses engaged and attuned, which reduces the potential for exteroceptive stimulation that is unexpected and therefore needlessly activating.

By doing a task or action over and over again, the neural pathways that are utilized begin to form systematic change within your brain. You can do that. The human brain seems to be built and programmed for upgrades at any time we choose. It is an available course. It's rhythm.

> The main point is that brain pathways can change as long as they are fired in certain scripted ways over an extended period of time. When fired together, the brain neurons begin to be wired together. The mind, then, becomes 'retooled' as a result (Kitayama & Park, 2010).

Predictability and routine may be the catalyst making compounded use of all mental wellness resources available to you.

RHYTHM IN PRACTICE

With growing knowledge and awareness, with insight into our identified values and desired direction, with a brain and body that thrives off rhythm, we can set the tempo on purpose. We repeat rhythms, forming new neural connections. We let the new pattern strengthen. Then, what began with intentional even painstaking trailblazing becomes the new norm. **We practice rhythm by building quality lifestyle patterns to foster and sustain mental wellness**.

Meditation Practice - A Guided Meditation of Connecting to Rhythm

As the circadian rhythm is a powerful clock for mental health, visualizing a connection to key points in a 24 hour period is beneficial to the brain. Go to kristaagler.com/book/keepinmind to listen to the provided audio

Table 10.1 *Cultivating a Rest Mentality*

Consider: When will you prioritize time for rest? What may need to be canceled or rescheduled to make space for rest? What do you notice of your mindset as you prioritize rest?			
Rest Time:	**Scheduled for:**	**What needs to move:**	**Observations:**
30 min/day			
4 hrs/week			
1 day/month			

or follow the accompanying prompts for a guided meditation pairing desired states with certain times of day, along with appropriate breathwork.

Reflection Practice – Cultivating a Rest Mentality

Take steps to punctuate your week and month with intentional rest, which is a movement away from taxing activity and toward activities that restore. Consider your mindset of rest: Do you view rest as an essential or a luxury? How might rest benefit you? When was the last time you rested on purpose? Do you allow and encourage others to rest?

Identify a new practice of rest to attempt and place it purposefully in the schedule. A possible starting point: try incorporating a 30 minute window of rest every day, a 4 hour window every week, and 1 full day each month, if that's available to you. You may have to make changes for this to be possible. Use Table 10.1 to prioritize time of rest. Observe what rest does for your brain and body.

Conscious Practice – Support Biological Rhythms

Modern life can set us out of time with our biological rhythms. However, as many of our systems can learn and adapt, we can take steps to bring our biological clocks back into rhythm. With awareness and adjustments, over time we will reap the benefits. Begin by checking in: Am I generally

Table 10.2 Support Biological Rhythms

Time Frame	Challenge	Support	Ease	Advantage
Circadian (24 hours)				
Circaseptan (7 days)				
Circalunar (30 days)				
Circannual (1 year)				

awake with the light and sleeping with the dark? Am I getting natural light as early in the day as possible? Are my daily patterns of eating, sleeping, and activity generally predictable?

Then, to expand whatever your current connection is to your biological rhythm, check in with the following four biological clocks: 24 hours (circadian), 7 days (circaseptan), 28 days (circalunar/infradian), and 1 year (circannual). Within each of these time frames, identify at least one time of challenge and at least one time of ease. Use Table 10.2 to note something that could support your system during the periods of challenge, and note an advantage available to you through the times of ease.

Lifestyle Practice – Establishing Rhythms of Predictability

Each day we have the simple opportunity to address our mental health by enhancing daily habits and implementing new, helpful patterns. Consider the things you do every day: Get out of bed. Brush teeth. Coffee. Shower. Dress. Greet roommate or partner or children. Drive or commute. And so forth. Consider all of your daily habits, then, begin with three, and consider how you could make those three activities work for you. What changes to that seemingly simple activity would make them more desirable or beneficial? What would make them more consistent with your values and desired direction? What would make them easier and streamlined?

Next, consider habits you would like to add to your daily life. Perhaps there are practices that don't have a place in your life currently, but that would benefit you. Zero in on three things you sense could make things just a bit better. Spend time mapping out the changes and putting any supports needed in place. Focus on implementing those changes slowly but surely, until they are lifestyle.

IN SUMMARY

Rhythm is essential for each human. As part of nature, the clockwork is built within us at a deep, genetic level. Remembering that we are rhythmic beings can illuminate uncomfortable shifts in our physical or psychological experience. It can then point us in the right direction of what work we need to do. Our well-being is shaped by a variety of biological clocks, from the well known circadian rhythm, to the lesser known circannual rhythm. Though there are general similarities of these clocks among humans, there is also nuance as to how each person functions biologically. With awareness of the biological clocks at play and mindfulness that pays attention to our own optimal functioning, we can make incremental changes for long term mental wellness.

REFERENCES

Asp, M. (2015). Rest: a health-related phenomenon and concept in caring science. *Global Qualitative Nursing Research, 2015,* 1–8.

Bilal, A., & Naveed, N. (2022). Biological rhythms, disorders and their energetic: a review. *Journal of Internal Medicine Research & Reports,* 1–4.

Blume, C., Garbazza, C., & Spitschan, M. (2019). Effects of light on human circadian rhythms, sleep and mood. *Somnologie, 23*(3), 147.

Coogan, A. N. (2013). Chronobiology and chronotherapy of affective disorders. *Journal of Cognitive and Behavioral Psychotherapies, 13*(1 A), 239–254.

Diddams, M., Surdyk, L. K., & Daniels, D. (2004). Rediscovering models of sabbath keeping: implications for psychological well-being. *Journal of Psychology and Theology, 32*(1), 3–11.

Foster, R. G., & Kreitzman, L. (2014). The rhythms of life: what your body clock means to you! *Experimental physiology, 99*(4), 599–606.

Fujiwara, H., Tsurumi, K., Shibata, M., Kobayashi, K., Miyagi, T., Ueno, T., ... & Murai, T. (2022). Life habits and mental health: Behavioural addiction, health benefits of daily habits, and the reward system. *Frontiers in Psychiatry, 13,* Article 813507.

Gu, Y., Gu, S., Lei, Y., & Li, H. (2020). From uncertainty to anxiety: how uncertainty fuels anxiety in a process mediated by intolerance of uncertainty. *Neural Plasticity,* Article 8866386.

Kitayama, S., & Park, J. (2010). Cultural neuroscience of the self: understanding the social grounding of the brain. *Social Cognitive and Affective Neuroscience, 5*(2-3), 111–29.

Kral, T. R. A., Imhoff-Smith, T., Dean, D. C., Grupe, D., Adluru, N., Patsenko, E., Mumford, J. A., Goldman, R., Rosenkranz, M. A., & Davidson, R. J. (2019). Mindfulness-based stress reduction-related changes in posterior cingulate resting brain connectivity. *Social Cognitive and Affective Neuroscience, 14*(7), 777–787.

Moreno, J. P., Crowley, S. J., Alfano, C. A., Hannay, K. M., Thompson, D., & Baranowski, T. (2019). Potential circadian and circannual rhythm contributions to the obesity epidemic in elementary school age children. *International Journal of Behavioral Nutrition and Physical Activity, 16*(1), 1–10.

Mutak, A., & Vukasović Hlupić, T. (2017). Exogeneity of the circaseptan mood rhythm and its relation to the working week. *Review of Psychology, 24*(1–2), 15–28.

Olejniczak, I., Pilorz, V., & Oster, H. (2023). Circle (s) of life: the circadian clock from birth to death. *Biology, 12*(3), 383.

Panda, D. S. (2020). *The circadian code. lose weight, supercharge your energy and sleep well every night.* Ebury Publishing.

Pengelley, E. (2012). *Circannual clocks: Annual biological rhythms.* Elsevier Science.

Proeschold-Bell, R. J., Stringfield, B., Yao, J., Choi, J., Eagle, D., Hybels, C. F., . . . & Shilling, S. (2022). Changes in sabbath-keeping and mental health over time: Evaluation findings from the sabbath living study. *Journal of Psychology and Theology, 50*(2), 123–138.

Raible, F., Takekata, H., & Tessmar-Raible, K. (2017). An overview of monthly rhythms and clocks. *Frontiers in Neurology, 8.*

Schulz, P. (2007). Biological clocks and the practice of psychiatry. *Dialogues in Clinical Neuroscience, 9*(3), 237–255.

Tan, Y., Van den Bergh, O., Qiu, J., & von Leupoldt, A. (2019). The impact of unpredictability on dyspnea perception, anxiety and interoceptive error processing. *Frontiers in Physiology, 10.*

Zhang, G., Chu, Y., Jiang, T., Li, J., Feng, L., Wu, H., Wang, H., & Feng, J. (2022). Comparative analysis of the daily brain transcriptomes of Asian particolored bat. *Scientific Reports, 12*(1).

PART III

COMMUNAL RESOURCES

Chapter 11

Gratitude: A Resource of Appraisal

Marc is a father whose children have grown, some having children of their own. Still, above all things, Marc is a father. He immigrated to the United States as a young man, quickly found work in construction and grew roots in the Midwest. He married in his twenties, and they quickly had five kids while he worked to become an electrician. In size and demeanor, Marc is solid, unmovable, stable.

His wife struggled with depression throughout her life, much like her father who died by suicide when she was seventeen. Navigating her depression was part of their family life. It was talked about, addressed, prioritized. Marc viewed caring for his wife's mental health like raising children and working his job: a duty and honor. When their youngest began to have similar struggles in her teenage years, they took it in stride. She battled depression until her death at age twenty-five.

Almost a year since she died, he thinks back on his daughter's last months, the things she said, the things she did. She died by her own hands and hid her plan to do so until the very end. In a statement that didn't make sense until after the funeral, she had told him that having him as a father was a reason to live. What seemed a sweet expression clarified in time as her beginning to say goodbye.

Marc sits in therapy, grave and undone by grief. His voice is an earthy bass, pronunciation soft, but clear. "You know, that is a gift. To be told that you were a reason to live through unspeakable pain for so long. She gave me that gift knowing what she would do." Then came a slow pause for a man who had already slowed to steady himself in the loss. "I carry that with me."

DOI: 10.4324/9781003521945-15

THE NATURE OF GRATITUDE

Gratitude gives room for grief and all else that's wrong. It finds a way to produce fruit out of good and hard alike. It may seem like an exercise in positivity, which really doesn't hold much water in the reality of life. Some hear the word "gratitude" and it seems dismissive of hardship. It's common that we hide the more painful parts of our lives, either from shame and embarrassment, or because others have responded poorly to attempts to be honest about the pain or discomfort in life. A flippant "be grateful" can be salt in the wound. The call to thankfulness may seem inappropriate, trite – even insulting or simply ineffective. Gratitude can be mistaken for a pleasing feeling when things go well. It can be oversimplified into a rote recitation of positive things, and although cataloging the good is a place to start, the full scope of the resource of gratitude lies well beyond that. It has applications for the full range of real life. In order for gratitude to function in a life that is often complex and difficult, it must contain depth and grit to match. If and when we look closely, we find that it does.

To deepen an understanding of gratitude, a single-lens approach is not ideal. Even in the field of psychology, there are varying perspectives. Some call gratitude an emotion, some a virtue of personality, and some a thoughtful choice. It is like the old story of six blind men approaching an elephant; one surmises he encounters a tree as he touches the leg, one suspects a rope as he grasps the tail, while a third insists it's a wall with two hands leaning against the immovable body, and so on (Reeves et al., 2007). Gratitude is understood by a variety of perspectives. All things considered, "gratitude is the positive recognition of benefits received" (Eid & Larsen, 2008), and such recognition takes place as a culmination of multiple capacities.

Gratitude is a resource of will-thought-emotion synergy, improving well-being in the practice of receiving good. The idea of gratitude is common, yet an assumption that we have a proper appreciation of it would be wide of the mark. It is a truly practical, holistic resource that engages our whole selves.

Gratitude involves emotion (a felt experience), thought (mental calculation), and will (choice). Together, these faculties can synthesize our experience of an unpredictable world so as to alter neural connections to increase well-being. Gratitude accomplishes all of the above through repetitive attempts at accepting the present positive realities.

Emotion – A Response to Gratitude

It may be important to note here that when I say "emotion," I mean the perceived experience or what is happening internally both psychologically and physiologically. The experience of emotion is distinct from the expression of emotion, which is the observable communication of what we call "feelings" (Metts & Planalp, 2011). Some would say of themselves "I'm not very emotional," and what they mean is that they are not very demonstrative of emotion. To be human is to have emotion-responsive experiences, though the expression can vary widely. When I talk of emotion, I am speaking of the resulting mental-physiological response to experience. So gratitude as an emotion is not a grin elicited or a contented sigh or a sunny giggle. It's not a fleeting "feeling." It's a substantial, brain-body experience that comes in response to acknowledging the good. "The virtue of gratitude is the willingness to recognize that one has been the beneficiary of someone's kindness, whether the emotional response is present or not" (Eid & Larsen, 2008). The neural mechanism of gratitude in the brain occurs whether or not there is an emotional expression. The shift in state is the emotion we are on the lookout for, not a reflexive feeling.

Gratitude is not smoothing over the unpleasant, brushing away the inconvenient, or suppressing suffering. It's opening eyes wider and applying attention more thoroughly in times when pain, disruption, or monotony move to take over our faculties. It's a thorough kind of honesty, requiring communication as well as acknowledgment of the good and hard the same (Algoe & Way, 2014). It challenges our brains, which are wired to identify threats over gifts.

Thought – An Appraisal Approach to Gratitude

The emotion involved in gratitude is not a function of reaction, and its role is not the desired end goal. We don't practice gratitude to feel good, and we don't wait until gratitude organically wells up within us. If gratitude includes emotion, then "gratitude is a feeling that depends on thinking" (Visser, 2012). Gratitude is, in part, a "form of subjective value," meaning that it is the result of the worth we ascribe to something (Yu et al., 2018).

Gratitude is not primarily a reflexive response to the situation, but is more shaped by our estimation of it; it is more selection than spontaneous. Though this means more work, it also means you do not have to be resigned to the joy your present circumstances seem to allow. Perhaps you can't just "be happy," but you can adjust your mental calculations about your situation with gratitude that ushers in well-being as well as pleasant emotions.

Some in the field of psychology call this view of gratitude the "appraisal approach" (Yu et al., 2018). The neuroscience is clear that the positive emotional experience comes on the tail end of specific ways of thinking about an experience, or what they call "cognitive antecedents." How we think about a situation is, in essence, our "appraisal" of it. It's the same idea of appraisal in buying or selling a house. The house will be appraised at a certain value based on its quality. Problems of disrepair in the house will be noted as well as assets. The appraised value is what the house appears to be worth. If you want to be sure the house is being appraised for the utmost value, you may get it reappraised. It's not to say that what is broken down in the house or what is in need of repair is not there, but it is to say that nothing of value is to be missed. So it is with gratitude; there may be some things wrong, maybe extensive disrepair, and yet there is the potential to reappraise the situation to not miss a single point of value.

We have the opportunity to approach specific aspects of our lives, or indeed our life as a whole, with similar reappraisal. Such "cognitive antecedents" are the thinking upon which gratitude depends. Gratitude is more than a positive emotional experience because we have something good. Any emotion stems out of roots of intentional cognitions that are, to a meaningful extent, within our control. "The emotional response is altered based on a reappraisal of the emotion-eliciting situation . . . the meaning of the situation is changed" (Boggio et al., 2019).

Will – Choosing Gratitude

Historically, gratitude has been seen as a virtue and ingratitude as a flaw. Researchers of gratitude mark the distinction by the choice to either acknowledge the good or not (Navarro & Tudge, 2020). Any context is a place for gratitude because it is not dependent on spontaneous reaction but on deliberate choice. It's a quiet resolution to acknowledge the good, to illuminate the remnant – even after loss. The good remaining after and within hardship matters more than it once did. Gratitude in adversity honors what was lost and can speak more loudly and justly of what has gone wrong. Gratitude is not trivializing the trauma; it is standing in the place of pain, and seeing all that remains. It simultaneously mourns the hurt while also tending to the vestige of what you once knew, nothing is taken for granted.

Since gratitude has a place in any context, it can become a trail between the darkest times to coming again to places of peace. In the neutral moments and in the really good days, the risk of missing the full experience comes not from the competition of pain but from complacency. Gratitude in the context of good and neutral times trains attention to value and receive what would otherwise be missed. It includes a conscious positioning of the self in any context to see good, acknowledge good, and receive good. It's a purposeful choice to tune in, pivot toward, look up to seek that which is alive, beautiful, brilliant, pure, kind, whole, creative, inspiring, soothing, welcoming, and fresh.

Our brains and bodies naturally brace to protect from the fall, the unexpected, the wave. We are used to that posture and we are built to not miss the threat and to prevent lack (Xavier de Lima et al., 2022). We could stay in that mode for the entirety of our lives. Or, we can shift slowly but surely and train our brain and bodies in becoming participant observers to the parts of our world that are good and right, right now. We orient ourselves as we direct ourselves by choice.

THE SCIENCE OF GRATITUDE

Universally helpful, gratitude is also practical, versatile for each person. It's not something that just works for some. It's not a way of mentally tricking yourself into thinking things aren't so bad. It functions within the brain to bring observable change and renaissance. **Gratitude provides a way to cause a shift at a neurological level for tangible improvement both in the moment and long term**.

A Paradigm Shift

Gratitude is part genetic expression. There is a genetic disposition where some are more naturally grateful than others; however, this is not set in stone. People have a "set point" of happiness, a general range of mood (Emmons, 2007). We have elevated emotions and we have low emotion states, but generally we come back to a "baseline" unique to ourselves. So there are those who seem to be happy all the time, who likely have a baseline of happiness that rides on the high side. Then there are those who seem to be unhappy no matter what, with a baseline on the low side.

Get this: A practice of gratitude raises that baseline, some research shows, by 25% (Emmons, 2007). That's a huge number. Imagine if in three months your income increased by 25%. Or what if your GPA improved by 25% by the end of next semester. Picture if you could run 25% faster, grow hair 25% thicker, sleep 25% longer, or whatever you want more of. We do a lot more for a lot less, and yet, gratitude remains woefully untried though it boasts the potential to give you a 25% happier baseline.

It takes time. At first, we benefit from a state of gratitude, which is temporary though real. Over time, we can develop trait gratitude, which is the point where it has become a way of life, increasingly part of one's personality. As we move along the spectrum from momentary experiences of gratitude to gratitude as a way of life, we increasingly improve our mental experience across the board. We increase our ability to regulate our experience of emotions, regardless of their nature (Boggio et al.,

2019). Anger, sadness, discontentment, jealousy, and the like begin to come more within our reign as we increase in gratitude.

The picture begins to take shape: gratitude is more than a flimsy attempt to feel better with glib positivity. Though potentially pleasant in its immediate practice, it activates deeper mechanisms in order to build a better psychology overall. It manifests wellness in our mental health, in our physical health, and in our relational health (Eid & Larsen, 2008). If there was a medication that did all that gratitude does, we would all be on it.

A Glance at the Neuroscience of Gratitude

Gratitude research discusses activity within the medial prefrontal cortex (mPFC) (Yu et al., 2018). It's not ideal to splice what different segments of the brain do as there's so much interplay, but at times in order to grasp a concept an oversimplifying breakdown is helpful. Within the mPFC central in mechanisms of gratitude, we have the ability to, among other things, understand our context and ascribe meaning to experiences and phenomenon. It's partially where we make sense of stimulus and attempt to relate adaptively to experiences.

Instinctively, our brain will use past experiences to orient ourselves to a situation. Depending on the context the brain fills around the situation, we may experience desire or threat or anything in between. A doctor's office could mean relief or concern. A stage could ignite thrill or terror. A car pulling into the driveway may evoke excitement or fear. Functioning within the mPFC determines the difference. The same situation with different framing changes not only my emotions but my physiological response as well. It's a function that we can sway toward our advantage by implementing gratitude. The shift can happen on a small, momentary scale, but can also be applied for widespread, overarching change to mindset.

The anterior cingulate cortex (ACC) is responsible for many functions: attention direction, threat scanning, error detection, reward seeking, among many others (Xavier de Lima et al., 2022). A thin section of this part of the brain is the pengual ACC (pgACC) and is the center for positive emotional experiences. It is also where gratitude overwhelmingly registers (Yu, et al., 2018). The overlap can be used for our advantage. Even though someone's natural baseline may not be prone toward positive emotional states, gratitude can be a direct line to that part of the brain.

An important message to reiterate here: the brain can change! It is adaptable, and one way we mold it is through use and repetition. The practice of gratitude, lighting up most in the pgACC, causes neural connections, encouraging active use and, therefore, enhancing a part of the brain highly connected to positive experiences of well-being and pleasant feelings (Yu et al., 2018). Furthermore, the stronger the representation of gratitude within the pgACC, the more that an individual will experience gratitude as a long-term trait rather than as merely a temporary state. Ongoing practice takes us from an experience to a way of being, from a moment to shaped identity.

Now, the ACC is responsible for, among other things, threat detection, or a scanning of the environment for any error we might make that could cost us. For our survival, we are more biased toward assessing threats. With that focus in the brain, our thoughts, emotions, and physiology are accordingly poised. The functioning of gratitude in the brain shifts us from threat-focus domination to make room to include benefit focus. The latter induces positive emotions, relaxed states, and subsequently, activation of favorable neural circuitry, impacting the extent of our human systems. The result can be reduced muscle tension and reduced inflammation responses (Hazlett et al., 2021), the effects of which are wide reaching.

The Cost and Benefit of Gratitude

Fascinatingly, the domain of gratitude does not stop with benefit, but includes and utilizes cost as well. Awareness of benefit and awareness of cost or threat cohabitate in the ACC portion of the brain. Cost awareness is a key part of gratitude, as gratitude is an awareness of receiving good almost always at some cost to another. Sometimes the cost is obvious: receiving an organ transplant, a flat tire changed on a rainy highway, eating a meal made by another's hands. Some cost falls beneath our notice: a spouse doing their part each day, a grocer steadily filling bags of food for a week, a friend offering a cup of coffee. More of our interactions involve cost than we notice, be it money, energy, effort, time, space, and so on. Most of the benefit we experience was served by someone at some point. The brain looking for threat, assessing what could cost us, also houses the component of pleasant well-being made possible by gratitude, recognizing our good at the cost of another. Sometimes the cost isn't what was directly paid but what others may be without. Gratitude for a sunrise may come at no expense to another human (though perhaps others made it possible for you to be in the position to enjoy it), but it is a sunrise not privileged to everyone. It is an experience lost to another, so gratitude, which includes an awareness of benefit by cost, applies here.

The neural function of gratitude does not just offer some balance to an overly attuned "error detector." It draws from that very awareness of cost and translates it into a deeper experience of receiving. In gratitude, we light up the pgACC, extracting well-being from what relates to threat or cost. "It seems therefore that a benefactor's cost may play a more prominent role in the generation of grateful feelings than the benefit one receives" (Yu et al., 2018). In other words, it's not the attaining that has the strongest impact; it's the awareness of the relationship between cost and benefit that makes gratitude so neurologically powerful. It's not having the thing that brings you joy; it's a recognition that you are receiving that thing at a cost somewhere along the line, usually by the kindness or generosity of another.

Gratitude is not the feel-good of getting what I want; it's an experience of receiving and an acknowledgement that the gift was made possible with a cost. This relationship of cost-benefit is important because it is the honesty to consider both of these in tandem that makes gratitude doubly powerful, beyond the delight of dwelling on the good. Using our control of thoughts for reappraisal is a crucial component of gratitude. That partnership changes the dynamic of potential in hardship. The cost and the benefit find a way of connecting, and the noticing and expressing of the benefit, even amidst great cost, results in an undeniable increase in mental well-being. (Yu et al., 2018). Practicing gratitude keeps us from forfeiting the remaining good in the aftermath of pain, trauma, or loss. Often the gratitude doesn't outweigh the suffering. However, it is a true and real good, the receiving of which elicits a measure of relief and an improvement through the whole system that allows for survival of the unimaginable. Deep suffering and loss is not a reason to pass by gratitude; rather, that's when gratitude is in its element.

The Result

So gratitude has its place in difficulty, and yet it offers to its practitioners a wealth of healing and protection. Highly grateful people, compared to their less grateful counterparts, tend to experience positive emotions more often, enjoy greater life satisfaction and more hope, and also tend to experience less depression, anxiety, and envy. They tend to be more empathetic, forgiving, helpful, and supportive as well as less focused on materialistic pursuits (Eid & Larsen, 2008).

As we grow in regular practice of gratitude, we inoculate ourselves against the worst effects of adversity, improve self-esteem, and increase confidence in life direction while simultaneously improving physical health at a generalized level (Wei et al., 2021). In our focus on available, accessible resources for mental wellness for everyone, it doesn't get much better than gratitude, which offers a holistic, widespread benefit through a neurological mechanism activated by you at any time.

GRATITUDE IN PRACTICE

We shift into a lifestyle of gratitude by practice. "We cultivate gratefulness by structuring our lives, our minds, and our worlds in such a way as to facilitate awareness of gratitude-inducing experiences and labeling them as such" (Eid & Larsen, 2008). The return on investment with gratitude is high from the outset. Even practicing as little as once a week boasts noticeable mental and physical health improvements. It seems gratitude functions with an innate ability to improve emotions, thought patterns, relationships, physical well-being, and general contentment, even after the first attempt. Though there are immediate effects, continued practice maintains the positive results. Research shows that after an intensive or ongoing period of gratitude practice, the benefits are still present six months after the practice and beyond (Eid & Larsen, 2008). It's that shift in "set point" or "baseline" that's transformative for long-term healing.

To have the capacity to desire nothing else in an imperfect moment or even a moment of pain is to wake up to the full-spectrum of your life that may only rarely be everything you want it to be. Gratitude connects us to vibrant life, with no conditions. **We practice gratitude by aligning will, thoughts, and emotions with the real and present good, even in hard times.**

Meditation Practice – A Guided Meditation on Setting a Course for Gratitude

Like tuning to a radio frequency, we can tune the brain and body to receive gratitude more readily and clearly. Through the following meditation, we will prime neural pathways to better practice and live with gratitude. Go to kristaagler.com/book/keepinmind to listen to the provided audio or follow the accompanying prompts for a guided meditation on posturing the whole self toward gratitude.

Reflection Practice – Enhancing "List" Gratitude

Begin a daily practice of gratitude with simple lists, repetition in pursuit of accumulation. Each day, intentionally make note of the good. Such "listing" is really the elementary level of gratitude; it's essential, though not the most difficult nor the most transformative of gratitude practices. It is a place to start. Go beyond using internal thought to express gratitude, making note of each source of good. Writing them down or speaking them out loud is important in externalizing the recognition and appreciation. The act of writing down what we're grateful for is demonstrated to improve beneficial outcomes (Boggio et al., 2019). Consider using Post-its on a wall, the boxes on a paper calendar, a note page on your phone, a text thread with others, a daily voice memo, a blank journal, a 3 x 5 card in your wallet, or any external method that comes to you.

Next, take steps to enhance the "listing" practice by doing so with a level of alert engagement maximizing neurological effects. There are many ways to wake up the brain-body system to best take in a gratitude practice. You could tune in to the five external senses: sight, hearing, taste, smell, and touch. You could also use movement such as stretching, a brief walk, or briskly rubbing your hands together for 20 seconds. You could also use an activating breath by shortening inhales and exhales, breathing in just for one second and immediately exhaling for one second for a total of about ten rounds.

With alert engagement, write responses to the following prompts. What are three present, positive realities today? What good or help did you receive today? What in your body, home, or life is working as it should, but may often go unnoticed until it's not working properly? Identify long-standing good things in your life that you've grown accustomed to and renew gratitude for their continued presence in your life.

Conscious Practice – The Essential Role of Story in Gratitude for the Brain

In the neuroscience of gratitude, practices most effective in creating change in neural circuitry involve stories. The part of the brain associated with the positive benefits of gratitude are activated by the progression of stories involving a few phases: (1) a need, problem, or deficit, (2) a fulfillment,

Table 11.1 *The Essential Role of Story in Gratitude for the Brain*

Prompt	Response
The Lack - Identify clearly the need, deficit, or struggle.	
The Gift - Identify the good, fulfillment, or support.	
The Response - Identify the expressed or appropriate appreciation, reception, or acknowledgment.	

a help offered, or a gift given, and (3) a response of emotion (the internal experience and not necessarily the impromptu expression) in receiving and appreciating (Fox et al., 2015). When we spontaneously experience gratitude, these are the dynamics at play. When we seek to intentionally practice gratitude, these are helpful components to prioritize.

Interestingly, the focusing on such story dynamics does not have to be limited to our own personal experience. You can experience gratitude at a neurological level by purposefully considering the gratitude narrative of another person (Fox et al., 2015). Neurologically, we practice gratitude by consciously reviewing the key elements of a story of receiving good that brought a desired change.

For this practice, consider a story of when needed help or good was received. It may be your own. It may belong to another. It may be from the news. Mindfully think through the three elements of gratitude narratives, and engage in interoception while responding in the space provided in Table 11.1. In daily life, look for these elements in any variety of contexts.

Table 11.2 *Gratitude Reappraisal*

Option 1 Script	Option 2 Script
"Even though [the difficulty] ____________________, I see/receive good in [the value/good] ____________________."	"If not for [the difficulty] ____________________, I would miss [the value/good] ____________________."
Example: "Even though this is a bad time for me to come down with the flu, I see value in the couch I am laying on and the rest I am forced to take."	**Example:** "If not for my son falling and skinning his knees, I would miss this opportunity to be close, comfort him, and show him I love him."
"Even though ____________________, I see/receive good in ____________________."	"If not for ____________________, I would miss ____________________."

Lifestyle Practice – Gratitude Reappraisal

By building the skill of reappraisal, or recalculating how we see our life to not miss any good or value, over time we positively change how we experience the reality of our lives. Gratitude in hard times is not about canceling out but about tuning in. Table 11.2 provides a couple sentence structures that can guide us in reshaping how we think about the hard aspects of life. Learning to use these scripts works in training neural networks to position ourselves for mental wellness, even in difficulty. The scripts are a reappraisal, both acknowledging the truth of the difficulty, but not leaving it at that.

Refer to Table 11.2. Identify a moderately difficult aspect of your current life. As this is a practice to train real-time thinking, I want to encourage you to not push yourself with the most painful parts of life. Consider reappraisal of the difficulty through use of these two sentence structures that acknowledge both the lack and the gift. The affliction is real; the consolation equally so. Gratitude aims not to miss the latter because of the former.

IN SUMMARY

Gratitude is a way of positioning the entire human system to feel better and live better. More than an emotional state, gratitude functions in a way that can be intentionally activated to promote change and well-being. Emotion is a facet of gratitude that at times feels pleasant and at other times is present as a neurological and biological shift that may not immediately connect with observable feelings. Thoughts can be selected to direct our awareness to the good, orienting the brain-body system in a more adaptive way. Choice is a key element of gratitude as it requires conscious engagement and selection. With emotion, thoughts, and choice working together, gratitude fires in the brain to produce holistic benefit. Your brain and body were wired to draw wellness from present positive realities even during pain and difficulty. Gratitude is available to each of us. It is transformative of the ordinary. As John Milton said, "gratitude bestows reverence, allowing us to encounter everyday epiphanies, those transcendent moments of awe that change forever how we experience life and the world" (2003).

REFERENCES

Algoe, S. B., & Way, B. M. (2014). Evidence for a role of the oxytocin system, indexed by genetic variation in cd38, in the social bonding effects of expressed gratitude. *Social Cognitive and Affective Neuroscience, 9*(12), 1855–1861.

Boggio, P. S., Giglio, A. C. A., Nakao, C. K., Wingenbach, T. S. H., Marques, L. M., Koller, S., & Gruber, J. (2019). Writing about gratitude increases emotion-regulation efficacy. *The Journal of Positive Psychology, 15*(6), 783–794.

Eid, M., & Larsen, R. J. (2008). *The science of subjective well-being.* Guilford Press.

Emmons, R. A. (2007). *Thanks!: How practicing gratitude can make you happier* (1st ed.). Houghton Mifflin.

Fox, G. R., Kaplan, J., Damasio, H., & Damasio, A. (2015). Neural correlates of gratitude. *Frontiers in Psychology, 6,* 1491–1491.

Hazlett, L. I., Moieni, M., Irwin, M. R., Haltom, K. E. B., Jevtic, I., Meyer, M. L., Breen, E. C., Cole, S. W., & Eisenberger, N. I. (2021). Exploring neural mechanisms of the health benefits of gratitude in women: a randomized controlled trial. *Brain Behavior and Immunity, 95,* 444–453.

Metts, S., & Planalp, S. (2011). Emotion experience and expression. In M. L. Knapp & J. A. Daley (Eds.), *Handbook of interpersonal communication* (pp. 283–315). Sage.

Milton, J. (2003). *Paradise lost.* Penguin Classics.

Navarro, J. L., & Tudge, J. R. (2020). What is gratitude? Ingratitude provides the answer. *Human Development, 64*(2), 83–96.

Reeves, N. P., Narendra, K. S., & Cholewicki, J. (2007). Spine stability: The six blind men and the elephant. *Clinical Biomechanics, 22*(3), 266–274.

Visser, M. (2009). *The gift of thanks: The roots, persistence, and paradoxical meanings of a social ritual.* Harper Perennial.

Wei, H., Hardin, S. R., & Watson, J. (2021). A unitary caring science resilience-building model: unifying the human caring theory and research-informed psychology and neuroscience evidence. *International Journal of Nursing Sciences, 8*(1), 130–135.

Xavier de Lima, M. A., Baldo, M. V. C., Oliveira, F. A., & Canteras, N. S. (2022). The anterior cingulate cortex and its role in controlling contextual fear memory to predatory threats. *Elife, 11.*

Yu, H., Gao, X., Zhou, Y., & Zhou, X. (2018). Decomposing gratitude: representation and integration of cognitive antecedents of gratitude in the brain. *The Journal of Neuroscience: The Official Journal of the Society for Neuroscience, 38*(21), 4886–4898.

Chapter 12

Village: A Resource of Relational Perception

"Everything, we do together." She said it not with nostalgia, as if referencing utopia, and not with annoyance, as if it was inconvenient. It was a matter-of-fact. Fatima tells stories of life in her home country in Eastern Africa. She tells of times spent around fires. She speaks of gathering around a plate of food, one large plate for many hands. She speaks of tasks being shared so that food preparation and washing and childcare are each a common task, not a list of jobs happening separately in each home.

Fatima came to the Midwest on refugee status. Her perilous journey is full, twisting, and against odds. As staggering and gripping as it is, her story is not rare but shared by many. Everything, we do together. She had been through a lot, lost too much. She had been in the United States, in the same house for almost eight years, when she began to speak of the grief of losing her village. She's gone through trauma therapy, and yet she struggles to feel herself.

"Here, everything is separate." She suspects it is the way of life here, disjointed and independent, that is in part to blame for her immovable sadness. The loss she's experienced, though felt, doesn't intimidate her. "We mourned together. What you lose, I lose. Now, the big and the small is mine alone. It is unbearable."

Unbearable. She speaks of a life to which many have grown accustomed, shirking interdependence and feeling proud to not need another. She knew better. Symbiosis was a fact of life. The common understanding of mutual dependence encouraged mutual investment. Fatima didn't want to find a way to feel better in a new norm of independence; she wanted her village back.

DOI: 10.4324/9781003521945-16

THE NATURE OF VILLAGE

Village is essential. It's nonnegotiable. To omit village is to shortchange mental wellness. That being said, village is not only found in deep, lifelong friendships. Indeed, those may be rare. Village, the real potential of the resource, is found in fluctuating measure with each intentional interaction between people.

The role of village in mental health may be different from what is coming to your mind now as you think of connecting with people. The people around you may or may not be compatible, helpful, or even close. That is not what the resource of village is about. Rather, it is interacting with others in a way within your control that empowers the brain to operate more vibrantly. The brain seems programmed to function within a social context. As we'll learn, there is an aspect of this that is not contingent on the number of relationships you have or even your particular enjoyment of them.

Village is the resource of regulating connection with the people within proximity, resulting in improved functioning and adaptive change. To be clear, the people around you are not in themselves the resource but rather the optimal functioning that we nurture at a brain level when we behave in a communal manner by connecting with each other. With this resource, we're not drawing from or using people; we're drawing from our brains in the lush context of human interaction.

WHAT MAKES A VILLAGE

Even though we will be discussing a lot of "social" and "relational" dynamics, the direction we are headed is not the surface of what's being said or felt in an interaction. Rather, in talking about connections between people, we are talking about connections within the brain and within your whole system. When I use the word "social," I mean that which is communal, interactive with other humans, in the way of living among others. And when I describe something as "relational," I simply mean the ways in which two or more people are connected.

Indeed, "social connections reach deep into the body to regulate some of our most fundamentally internal molecular processes" (Eisenberger & Cole, 2012). It's part of basic functioning, not just at an awareness level but at a molecular level, the basic building blocks of each human being. There are mountains of information and research on the effects of any number of social or relational dynamics on mental health. Our focus is narrow: the available dynamics of the people around you that can be tapped by your choice for your brain and body to function more as it seems it was meant to, for your mental wellness. Such a narrow approach will leave out much of what impacts you in your relationships. It's a resource that's available to all, but one that can tend to get away from us.

When it comes to mental health, there is increasing concern of exchanging real, valuable person-to-person contact in favor of a mirage-like experience of imitation connection.

> The twenty-first century has unleashed a tsunami of opportunities for social engagement and accelerated the flow of social information. Yet as our outlets for social sustenance proliferate, along with the global population, there is a paradoxical increase in social isolation within society. The proportion of the population who live alone has risen and an increasing number of people experience loneliness (Matthews & Tye, 2019).

The impression is that we are more connected than ever; the reality is that we are essentially more secluded. Returning to a village frame of mind is essential to brain health and mental wellness.

The word "village" technically means a gathering of houses that is smaller than a "town" and implies a group of people with shared space (Evers, 2023). In essence, it is a term that sketches out limits to a community within which there is knowable potential. In other words, the village is a group of people defined by the capacity for interaction. It is encapsulated by the circle tracing the limits of our social span.

Dunbar's Number is a widely referenced estimation that we can keep up healthy relationships with around 150 people, based on a study done on primates. Fascinatingly, similar research done on humans reveals no such predictable number. The range is wide, between 4 and 290 people, depending on the person being studied (Lindenfors et al., 2021). What this means is that for some people, maintaining 4 relationships is the limit of how many people they can beneficially and sustainably maintain connection, while others can manage almost 300. Each of us has a different, unique capacity for villages of differing sizes. Again, the presence of bio-individuality is worth noting, so your role is to pay attention to your own functioning rather than getting your cues of how to function socially by comparison with others.

You may have an idea of how many people with whom you can engage in an authentic relationship and sustain it for a long period of time. Alternatively, that may be an area in which you need to cultivate some awareness. Village refers to the unique optimal range of human interaction specific to you. It is worth noting, relatively few relationships can be an effective village. The more is not necessarily the merrier. As we'll find, the indicator of how your village positively impacts your mental health is not in the number of people or even in the actual experience of those relationships.

We understand and orient ourselves in part through the feedback loops of our "close-others" (Courtney & Meyer, 2020). It's how we establish our place and footing. We pace our mental and emotional effort, time invested, and the degree to which we draw near to others based, uniquely, on where we find ourselves within a social constellation. It matters how we view it, and doing so mindfully is to our advantage. Rather than quantity, and even beyond quality, it is the way in which we approach and think of our village that provides mental wellness.

Risks and Advantages of Village

In researching the correlation with social health and mental health, the connection is well established. In our earliest development as babies and children, our brains experience more pervasive and complex learning when done in relationship. "We are shaped by other people and crave for social contact to the extent that isolation is used as punishment and even as torture. According to a recent meta-analysis, social isolation and loneliness are risk factors for increased mortality" (Hari et al., 2015). To be disconnected from people in a meaningful way runs a risk to mental and physical health. We hold the capacity to turn the tide of that force. As isolation can cause damage, connection can breed life and wellness.

From enjoyment of life to experiences of vitality, the benefits of village are many. "Socially connected individuals live longer and show increased resistance to a variety of somatic diseases ranging from heart disease to cancer" (Eisenberger & Cole, 2012). Neural circuitry, hormone regulation, immunity, disease response, and systemic inflammation all respond to the ebbs and flows of our social connection. It cannot be ignored; one way or another, how you relate to the people around you is, in fact, shaping your mental wellness.

Perhaps, for you, the idea of other people being a pivotal force in your life causes you to bristle a bit. Perhaps it's been a source of frustration or of absence or of hurt. The work at hand is to acknowledge where we lack this resource and then turn our attention to what is available to us. Too often, I have seen the hurt caused by a few keeping a person from the many at hand. It can be nerve-racking to move out of the ways you've learned to protect yourself from people, and it can be challenging to reshape long-held habits that no longer serve us. Even so, mindful forward movement is necessary as your mental wellness may be improved or capped by your approach to the village resource.

There are risks in relationships, and not just hurt and disruption, but also in a very real activation of the threat response in our systems (Porges, 2003). We need to approach this resource very specifically. It's not a goal of meeting more people or being more social. The approach we take and how we view real-life interactions with others is the key. Relationships are hard, and yet we need them. We are wired for survival, and this can draw us both toward the village, and can cause us to run from people. "The paradox underlying much of the push-pull ambivalence in human relationships is that we are wired both for self-protection and for connection" (Fishbane, 2007). The resource of village is not mastery of that push-pull. It is a mindset that ensures we position ourselves with the village around us in a way that serves survival. Our approach can initiate healing change from the molecular to the neurological to the physiological, indeed to your whole life.

Willingness: The Point of Entry

As the resource of village is open to the influence of others' actions, the path here is anything but direct. Thankfully, our access to village does not require mastery, ease, or likeability. Simple willingness and attendance do the trick. Our brain-body system stands ready to make use of the human connection available around us. Our past experience with people is a factor, but not a make-or-break one. "The tone is one of acceptance and curiosity about one's own experience, rather than a repressive attempt to control one's reactivity" (Fishbane, 2007). In approaching other people, we gain and contribute most (from a mental health standpoint) when we pay attention to the interaction and to ours and the others' response in the interaction. The goal is not a specific feeling or experience but a heightened tuning in from which we learn more, grow more, and are more available for others to do the same. It is showing up for the bidirectional exchange that happens imperceptibly between people for our mutual benefit. It is a brain and body shift in real terms.

THE SCIENCE OF VILLAGE

The brain, it seems, is built in a way that requires social engagement to work properly and avoid decline (Felix et al., 2021). And yet, it would seem cruel that arguably the most vital organ in our bodies could be so dependent on the influence of other people. Thankfully, that's not how it works. What we will find is that although relational connection reaches throughout our brains and bodies, the primary factor of how that happens is a mechanism within our control. Like a single-handled faucet that runs both hot and cold water, we possess a lever of sorts that can change the "temperature" of social influence. Before identifying that powerful lever, some background is important.

Discussions of neuroscience or parts of the brain serve to help us see the work we do as very real and directly influential. In as much as other people are "out there," we might be tempted to externalize the mechanism. The primary influence is not from the outside working in or others' actions shaping our mental wellness. The primary change agent is within our purview, in the jurisdiction of our own brains. **Village provides needed stimulation and context with which the brain is better suited to pursue mental wellness.**

The Village, the Brain, the Nervous System

The brain belongs in a communal setting. Certainly not every social setting, and not at all times, but as we exist in a world with necessary sunshine, water, and food, we require regular doses of human contact. It is part of the survival functioning innate in humans and shapes the development of many essential skills (Nelson et al., 2016). From birth throughout life and through old age, relationships are needed for the brain to develop and for neurons to function (Fishbane, 2007). The brain will deteriorate without the firing and lighting up that happens through relational interaction. The neural circuitry throughout our brain and bodies is reliant on the attention and imperceptible feedback we provide one another. The correlation is not a distant one. "Human connections create neuronal connections" (Siegel, 1999). Social interaction is crucial, mandatory in the functioning and healing of the brain.

Some studies of the brain reveal that thought patterns within our minds are more conversant than reflective. In other words, "humans are 'designed' for dialogs rather than monologues" (Hari et al., 2015). Beneath our conscious awareness, interacting with one another synchronizes some portion of thought and language, dispersing the "cognitive load" in the shared exchange. Often, even when alone, we think in internal conversations, indicative of the communal nature of our systems. The use or disuse of village causes widespread ramifications (Beutel et al., 2017).

Our social ties impact many regions of the brain: threat and alarm systems, safety, reward systems, the nervous system (Eisenberger & Cole, 2012). The teeter-totter of the nervous system, with its capacity to sound the alarm and its capacity to hit the snooze button, is intermittently activated in our social interactions.

Our brain-body connection seems to have no doubt that we need people, whether that be for meeting basic needs or for the brain to be healthy or anything in between. It responds seriously to experiences of availability of the resource as well as to lack. "To the extent that social connection is another critical ingredient for survival, experiences of social disconnection and connection may have co-opted this basic harm and reward circuitry, respectively" (Eisenberger & Cole, 2012).

When we have interactions of a positive nature, the parasympathetic nervous system is activated, grounding us in a brain-based experience of calm. The research points to these favorable exchanges bringing more activity to the brain regions associated with belonging and security while simultaneously reducing activity in the amygdala, that region known for hosting the alarm system (Eisenberger & Cole, 2012). Naturally occurring opioids in the body as well as oxytocin (feel good chemicals) are released in the body as a result of such interactions resulting in stress reduction.

It's a two-way street. Just as interactions that reinforce our connection to humanity bring calm, interactions that seem to threaten our attachments bring alarm and all the physiological responses that go with it (Eisenberger, 2013). The list is long of chronic, inflammation-related illnesses correlated with isolation (Smith et al., 2020). Inflammation is linked with mental disturbance as well. Real is the domino effect of social disruption, sympathetic nervous system activation, disease, and mental illness. An experience of social rejection can instigate a response similar to a survival threat (Tomova et al., 2021). An experience of social connection can initiate physiological responses consistent with abundance, safety, and well-being. The capacity to regulate the differing experiences of social connection or disconnection is the leverage our brain holds to utilize this resource.

PERCEPTION: OUR POWER IN CONNECTION

Here is where it gets interesting. The shift happening in the brain is based on the "subjective experience of social disconnect" (Eisenberger, 2013). Our subjective ideas, or our ideas shaped by our own interpretation, direct the nervous system in how to respond to a social interaction. It's not the interaction or context itself that is most impactful; it's our perception of it. In fact, our subjective or perceived impression of our social standing has a larger impact on our stress response and health than the objective or actual fact of our social situations (Eisenberger, 2013). How I think about my interactions with people is more influential than my actual level of connectedness or isolation. In other words, how I choose to interpret my social context is the deciding factor. In fact, "a large literature has developed showing that *perceived* social isolation in normal samples is a more important predictor of a variety of adverse behavioral, psychological, and health outcomes than objective isolation" (Cacioppo & Cacioppo, 2012).

Say you had spent time a couple continents away from a loved one, perhaps from Stockholm, Sweden to Buenos Aires, Argentina. On the return flight, you stop in Chicago to change flights. The distance is greatly reduced, and yet still sizable. The distance from Chicago to Stockholm is what it is. However, you can view it as "close" to your loved one, as your perception considers the closing of the distance. It could also be viewed through the hours still left to travel, and the perception could be that they are still far away. The distance is the same. Perception, which can be intentionally carved, shifts the experience.

The distinction between perception of connectedness and the quantity or quality of social connection is significant. It's the reason why village can be a mental health resource available to all. Admittedly, we have varying access to and different qualities of relationships, and much of that may be out of our control. Still, perception is a mechanism of control available in each of us. We may not be able to change the people around us or our social standing with any unilateral effect; however, we can certainly change our perception, and that is the power to change our mental wellness through this resource of how we connect with others. Reclaiming our perception is putting our hand on the lever, transforming how we draw from the resource of village.

It goes both ways. Whether my perception is toward connectedness or toward disconnection will determine the effects on my brain, body, and life.

> Perceived social support or social connection (the perception that one is cared for, loved and valued by others) predicts better health outcomes, whereas loneliness or social disconnection (the perception that one is socially isolated or not connected to others) predicts poorer health outcomes (Eisenberger & Cole, 2012).

To take some of the pressure off, it's not either-or. Like water temperature in the shower, there is a gradient at play that we can move along. "A person's position along the continuum of perceived social isolation/bonding to others is associated with a variety of physical and mental health effects" (Cacioppo & Cacioppo, 2012). These effects, among other things, include mood regulation, viral immunity, and regulation of inflammation as well as sleep quality and maintenance of energy.

Perception can increase in momentum, initiating an "interpersonal expectancy effect." In this, we begin orienting ourselves to our expectations, increasing the likelihood of experiences that match or are in alignment with our expectations. The research paints a picture of perception shaping not only the current social experience but also the lens through which we view future social interactions (Cacioppo & Cacioppo, 2012). So those who feel socially rejected by perception will demonstrate memory patterns increasingly inline with that perception, while those who focus on the connection they actually do experience will shape memory patterns that anticipate and therefore experience more connection.

Those with higher reports of loneliness, or more of a "perceived gap between the self and others," will report more similar experiences and also tend to see themselves in terms of similarity with others (Courtney & Meyer, 2020). Though it may seem intuitive to do so, when connection is contingent on similarity, then what makes me different can become a perceived threat to my well-being. It seems in drawing most optimally from your "village," it's important to note that difference does not have to equal distance, and that is the work of conscious perception. For mental wellness, difference can be observed and appreciated, closing the perception of distance between ourselves and others.

The Village in Front of You

The situation may seem risky if the value of relationships is tied to a specific number, a certain quality, an ability to charm, an availability, or a feel-good experience. None of those things you can guarantee, which would make the offering of village potentially quite scarce. But, if the scene is one where you can take whatever human contact is available to you and through your own faculties draw some measure of connection, then the entire landscape changes.

It is of serious relevance that social mental health benefits are not dependent on having best friends. "Social network research emphasizes the 'strength of weak ties,' specifically highlighting the important role acquaintances play in well-being, social support, and access to information" (Courtney & Meyer, 2020). It's not about the inner circle. It's awareness and engagement with whoever is before us.

We "map" our place within our social constellations. Our mapping involves perception, that we can consciously use to move from an experience of isolation to one of bonding. The number of people does not have to be large. Difference is not an obstacle, and distance is not ultimately a problem. We can select thoughts and approach our map in a way that highlights connection with our village, which includes a mindful number of people from the person closest to us to those "weak ties" with whom intentional interactions are still profitable for mental wellness.

The village becomes the person in front of you. There will be exceptions, but by and large, as we give attention to the people in our actual proximity with a mind to find contact, connection, and closeness, we will utilize village. How you approach a person is more important than who they happen to be. "During social interaction, people receive both conscious and unconscious social cues from others' expressions, gestures, postures, actions, and intonation. Thus, they automatically align at many levels, starting from bodily synchrony to similar orientations of interests and attention" (Hari et al., 2015). To tune in to others, we begin with mindfulness and direct that nonjudgmental, observational attention toward the other. Eye contact, which forms a sort of neurological loop between two people, is one way to choose connection (Fishbane, 2007). Interoception can include the nuanced awareness of what is going on within another person through these biological markers. We participate in a bidirectional interoceptive attunement with the goal of increased connection that comes with paying attention. Part of the experience of this intentionality we will be very aware of, while elements of it will fall beneath our consciousness while still shaping our brain-body experience of being with others.

VILLAGE IN PRACTICE

As a human, you are equipped to engage with other humans in a way that, although unique to you, is beneficial to you. The brain is not contingent on the fair weather of your current social context. Within your human system, you have what you need to draw deeper mental wellness. The obstacles are worth overcoming. To say otherwise would be to reinforce the damaging narrative that you are destined for isolation or that such aspects of your mental wellness are beyond your control. On the contrary and from the research, there is a clear benefit to prioritizing connection with others. **We practice village through intentionally approaching people and adjusting perception**.

Meditation Practice – A Guided Compassion Meditation

Practices of compassion toward others bring about an observable shift in internal experience. In focusing on the work of owning our perception of our connection to other people, compassion is a strategic place to begin. The provided meditation helps shape the brain's way of perceiving people, improving our sense of connectedness. Go to kristaagler.com/book/keep-inmind to listen to the provided audio or follow the accompanying prompts for a guided compassion meditation.

Reflection Practice – Shaping a Perception of Connectedness

With your daily life in mind, consider: Where do you see yourself on a spectrum between connected and isolated? Which direction do you lean? Your view of yourself on the spectrum impacts your mental wellness, yet is subject to change.

It does not matter how many friends you have or how close you feel to them. It does not matter how much people like you or how often you get together. What matters is how you choose to think about the relationships available to you today. In not being able to completely control your social life, you are still able to draw deep from the village well. Use Table 12.1

***Table 12.1** Shaping a Perception of Connectedness*

Prompt	Response
Where have you experienced safety, comfort, or acceptance in relationships? Note a time that you were able to provide these experiences for another.	
Where have you experienced honesty, support, and help in relationships? Note a time you were able to provide these experiences for someone else.	
Consider three central relationships in your life right now. Take time to note the aspects of those relationships that are collaborative, intimate, enjoyable. Be specific.	
In a typical day, where are you most likely to encounter strangers or acquaintances? Note the possible points of contact involved: eye contact, communication, etc. What might it be like to approach those encounters with mindful attention, senses engaged, or with a lens of your values?	

to reflect on your current relationships with people, from those you live with to acquaintances. Consider them in terms of how close they are to you rather than how far, how available they are rather than how unapproachable. Consider how differences are not obstacles to connection. In each question, the focus is on the amount, small or large, that is present of what we want to experience in our relationships. The degree to which interactions aren't beneficial is not the concern. It's as if we are using binoculars to zero in on any and all good that's present in all social exchanges.

Conscious Practice – Practicing Village by Practicing Gratitude

We can create authentic connection, even without intimacy. Think of times you've come together with strangers at a site of crisis. Or perhaps at a movie or concert, when laughter or cheering connected you with other audience members. One avenue for building connection is gratitude. The hormone oxytocin that is an active component of gratitude (Algoe & Way, 2014), is also the key hormone at play in attachment (Fishbane, 2007). It encompasses feeling safe and connected and facilitates states of calm connection. As the benefits of connection with people are vast and absolutely necessary, and the availability of quality, deep relationships is not always a guarantee, how wonderful that we can cultivate experiences of deep connection through gratitude.

Gratitude encourages ongoing engagement and receptivity between people, growing the relationship little by little (Algoe & Way, 2014). The positive chemicals activated in the brain also encourage both asking for help and extending it, further deepening connection and belonging (Eisenberger & Cole, 2012). The focus, then, for this practice is twofold.

First, ask for help and extend help. One component of gratitude is a need being met. We can encourage gratitude within our relationships by proliferating opportunities for needs to be met. Ask for help, large or small. Extend help, wherever you can. Right now, identify one request you could make of someone else. Then, identify one offer of help you have to give. Providing and receiving help is an avenue to connection, not to be missed.

Second, identify and express gratitude directly to others. No shortcuts. Simple and true appreciation spoken in person welcomes that shift in the brain, altering perception and experience. Even now, write down three names to begin taking the practice seriously. Identify who you have witnessed meet even small needs for you or for others, and verbally express it.

Lifestyle Practice – Seek to Notice the People Around You

Engage, in the present with your senses, with the person in front of you. Approach people with mindfulness. Begin a shift where most of your interactions with people, whether the stranger handing you your change or the partner you share a bed with, are rooted in mindful intent. Williams and Penman describe mindfulness with five points: paying attention, on purpose, to the present moment, without judgment, to the things that actually are (2011). These points can guide our interactions.

Pay attention by giving focused attention and tuning your senses to the other person. Engage on purpose, presenting your posture, facial expression, words, and listening to the living person before you. Be in the present moment, giving more of your mental and emotional energy to what is happening now than to history or what's next. Approach without judgment in that you aren't having to determine if aspects of the exchange are "good" or "bad"; simply notice the reality of the interaction. Relate to what actually is, gently refraining from responding to assumption, quick interpretations, or blind filling in of the gaps; allow more of your thoughts and emotions to reflect the facts of the exchange.

Perhaps approaching each interaction mindfully comes readily to you and reading the above is primarily a reminder. Perhaps such focused attention with people feels either foreign or intimidating. For the latter, begin by practicing three times this week. Looking at the coming days, pick three interactions you know you will have, such as buying coffee from the barista, a meeting with your boss, or taking care of a family member. For one interaction at a time, focus on the five points of mindfulness: Pay attention. On purpose. Present moment. Nonjudgment. Actual reality. Afterward, note what the experience was like.

A challenge for all of us: when going into an interaction with someone who is hard for you, use the same mindfulness points. Perhaps they annoy you, perhaps they've hurt you, or maybe they stand for something with which you seriously disagree. Being mindful in interactions is not about liking or agreeing; it is about being present and available to the exchange.

IN SUMMARY

It all comes down to a few points: Be mindful of the unique and optimal size of your social circle. This is your village. Help those people and ask them for help. Engage in gratitude in reflection and in expression. Most of all, be intentional to prioritize perception of the bonding you do experience and of the closeness available to you. This moves the brain from a disconnected threat state to a safe and connected state. This is how we position ourselves for the mental health benefits of being a human among humans. Drawing from village means owning how we approach person-to-person interaction. We are free from the goal of having a certain type of experience or emotional reaction. The mental health benefits of community in this perspective are not that they make us happy or meet our needs, though that happens at times. The mental wellness draw is that with other people our brain orients itself to the world around us, connects within itself more effectively, and experiences positive brain-body chemistry in the process of engaging.

REFERENCES

Algoe, S. B., & Way, B. M. (2014). Evidence for a role of the oxytocin system, indexed by genetic variation in cd38, in the social bonding effects of expressed gratitude. *Social Cognitive and Affective Neuroscience, 9*(12), 1855–1861.

Beutel, M. E., Klein, E. M., Brähler, E., Reiner, I., Jünger, C., Michal, M., ... & Tibubos, A. N. (2017). Loneliness in the general population: prevalence, determinants and relations to mental health. *BMC psychiatry, 17,* 1–7.

Cacioppo, S., & Cacioppo, J. T. (2012). Decoding the invisible forces of social connections. *Frontiers in Integrative Neuroscience, 6.*

Courtney, A. L., & Meyer, M. L. (2020). Self-other representation in the social brain reflects social connection. *The Journal of Neuroscience: The Official Journal of the Society for Neuroscience, 40*(29), 5616–5627.

Eisenberger, N. I. (2013). Social ties and health: a social neuroscience perspective. *Current Opinion in Neurobiology, 23*(3), 407–413.

Eisenberger, N. I., & Cole, S. W. (2012). Social neuroscience and health: neurophysiological mechanisms linking social ties with physical health. *Nature Neuroscience, 15*(5), 669–674.

Evers, J. (Ed.).(2023). *Village.* National Geographic Education.

Felix, C., Rosano, C., Zhu, X., Flatt, J. D., & Rosso, A. L. (2021). Greater social engagement and greater gray matter microstructural integrity in brain regions relevant to dementia. *The Journals of Gerontology: Series B, 76*(6), 1027–1035.

Fishbane, M. D. K. (2007). Wired to connect: neuroscience, relationships, and therapy. *Family Process, 46*(3), 395–412.

Hari, R., Henriksson, L., Malinen, S., & Parkkonen, L. (2015). Centrality of social interaction in human brain function. *Neuron, 88*(1), 181–193.

Lindenfors, P., Wartel, A., & Lind, J. (2021). "Dunbar's number" deconstructed. *Biology Letters, 17*(5).

Matthews, G. A., & Tye, K. M. (2019). Neural mechanisms of social homeostasis. *Annals of the New York Academy of Sciences, 1457*(1), 5–25.

Nelson, E. E., Jarcho, J. M., & Guyer, A. E. (2016). Social re-orientation and brain development: An expanded and updated view. *Developmental Cognitive Neuroscience, 17,* 118–127.

Porges, S. W. (2003). Social engagement and attachment: a phylogenetic perspective. *Annals of the New York Academy of Sciences, 1008*(1), 31–47.

Siegel, D. (1999). *The developing mind: How relationships and the brain interact to shape who we are.* Guilford Press.

Smith, K. J., Gavey, S., RIddell, N. E., Kontari, P., & Victor, C. (2020). The association between loneliness, social isolation and inflammation: A systematic review and meta-analysis. *Neuroscience & Biobehavioral Reviews, 112*, 519–541.

Tomova, L., Tye, K., & Saxe, R. (2021). The neuroscience of unmet social needs. *Social Neuroscience, 16*(3), 221–231.

Williams, M., & Penman, D. (2011). *Mindfulness: An eight-week plan for finding peace in a frantic world.* Rodale Books.

Chapter 13

Soul: A Resource of Consciousness Beyond Brain and Body

Walking on the red dirt of Western Tanzania, a group of women work to rebuild their lives within a refugee camp. Through microfinancing, they obtained sewing machines and they put them to good use, creating products, then finding unique ways to market and sell their goods beyond the camp. As they share the tasks of livelihood, washing and making food and such, they also share their load of grief. They reach out to one another, and as they each express the lack in what they have to give, together they reach beyond themselves.

In the evenings, as the sunset makes silhouettes of trees and tents and small buildings made of mud brick, they take time sharing their stories, fully and explicitly. Each has their turn, availing themselves of the chance to be fully heard. No rushing. One by one, a woman takes a seat in the middle and begins, "I will tell you my story. I will share with you my secrets." There is an open understanding that the hardship each of them has faced contains qualities of such intimacy and vulnerability, that their entire stories are worthy of secrecy. And yet, here they are, sharing them. Stories of loss, stories of separation, stories of violence.

Toward the end, one woman comes forward, and as she stands, total silence falls on the group. She comes to the center, falls to her knees, and with her head thrown back, she cries out with wailing sobs. The other women look on, many with silent tears, chins held up in respect. The unspoken is understood: of all they have suffered, this woman has walked through terrain more severe and unspeakable than the rest. They offer agreement and a communal holding. And there is not a word spoken.

When she finally stands, all stand with her. One woman begins drumming, and then another. It is not a sad drumming, not a rhythm of sorrow. And it is not a battle march, driven by anger. It's the percussion of spring,

DOI: 10.4324/9781003521945-17

rain on dry, dusty ground. The prismatic dresses of the women begin to swirl with their movement, and the group dances together in worship and prayer and a belief in life currently denied them in their physical brains, bodies, and location. Through their songs and surrender, they approach and enter an animating, comforting connection transcending place, time, and understanding. They would tell you: they are drawing from the soul.

THE NATURE OF SOUL

According to a Gallup Poll done in 2022, 81% of Americans believe in God (Jones, 2022). Although this is the lowest rate on record, it's significant that most Americans looking to improve their mental wellness likely have a belief in God and yet may not actively connect the two. When addressing physical or mental health, leaving out a person's spiritual or religious beliefs is documented as having a negative effect on well-being (Verghese, 2008). Since most adults report some kind of spiritual belief and there is documented proof of its benefit, it is not only clinically indicated to explore the role of spirituality in mental health, it is also compelling and worthwhile.

The goal here is to consider and frame belief as a spiritual reality, the functionality of which leads to improved mental health. Just as a placebo effect requires some actual belief to create an actual change of experience (Leibowitz et al., 2019), a willingness to actually attempt a belief in something beyond you is required for the mental health benefits we are targeting with the resource at hand. Faith traditions and assemblies may hold polarizing stimuli for different people, some holding great affection for their faith history and some deeply wounded from their exposure. Soul is the real, living capacity for spirituality within you that exists regardless of the positive or negative experiences you've had with religion.

I will draw from research reports, highlighting the data inferring the presence of the soul, as well as the research exhibiting its effective role in mental health. The pursuit of soul, for all its nuance and intangibility, is seen to invoke relief and measures of healing. Regardless of whether or not you consider yourself a spiritual person, I invite you to consider afresh this resource of soul.

The soul is "the immaterial essence and spiritual/animating principle embodied in human beings" (Merriam-Webster, n.d.). The Greek word for soul, "psyche," indicates breath and life, or the essential force, animating the brain-body system. For our discussion of soul as a resource, I would define soul as the incorporeal, living inner self that functions within and beyond our physical nature. It is, in many ways, unobservable in that it is not predominantly understood through direct observation, though indirect aspects of it are discoverable.

To consider the soul, we are considering the part of us that is not restricted to the physical body and brain. Though it is often approached through our physical understanding and capacities, it is the part of us that also somehow extends beyond those limits. **Soul is the resource of the part of humans able to exist beyond the confines of brain and body that benefits the whole system in ways not otherwise available.** In the coming pages, I will share just some of the research and insights from neuroscience on these aspects of the self that may exist beyond the brain and body. As all the various definitions above indicate, it is alive, dynamic, and invigorating to our humanity. It is both distinct from the physical while also presented and expressed within our physical self.

Distinguishing Soul

The history of the scientific quest to uncover the soul is fascinating. For hundreds of years, the best and brightest minds have tried to quantify and observe the elusive soul. Some have tried to weigh the body the instants before and after death in attempts to capture the weight of the soul, while others have taken photos of the same moments seeking any observable data. From early philosophers to renaissance scientists and modern neurosurgeons, humanity has sought to find it, to prove it, to disprove it (Pandya, 2011). With its liminal qualities that eclipse observation, consensus on what it is or if it in fact exists will remain elusive, especially in the world of science.

Conceptually speaking, "soul" is a term we use to describe what is unique to humanity and what cannot be broken down in a person, even as body or personality may break down. The soul is "resident within, but distinct from the human body" (Pandya, 2011). Soul implies essence, and speaks to the ubiquitous experience of being more than the output of biological, social, and physical mechanisms (Southwick et al., 2016). When we consider the soul as a valid, essential component of the brain-body-soul triad, the view of personhood, life, and living is necessarily altered.

Though the conversation of the existence of the soul is not new, it is indispensable for the work of mental well-being, particularly with one specific consideration. I have known, loved, and worked with individuals with brain injury. The damage can cause a number of disruptions, including to personality. I've seen the ensuing changes be at times troubling and painful, and I've seen the changes to personality seem pleasant, even improving relationships. All that to say, the damage to the brain and the subsequent loss to experience or personality may change much, but I would argue that there is a deeper essence of who that person is that remains regardless. Even in lieu of brain injury, humans may sustain other forms of harm that leave lasting damage to one's very identity. To defend the idea of soul is to defend the personhood of those whose body and brain cannot be the defining display of who they are, unique and valuable.

Brain, Body, and Soul

Shortly after its birth, the field of psychology began separating the brain from the body, giving it perhaps necessary individualized attention. Psychology became a branch of science distinct from the medical care of the body. Currently, many are making movements to bring those back together with a more holistic focus. Similarly, though the emergence of the field of psychology initially championed the study of soul, it eventually also separated it from the mind (Luccio, 2013). Psychologists and spiritual directors, therapists and clergy were designated in different roles and encouraged to stay in their lane. In many ways, it's been an appropriate distinction for providers to stay within their areas of expertise, but the point remains: There was a time when the mind and the body and the soul were not seen as separate. All were seen to be real, to be connected, and to be needed. As the fields of psychology and medicine continue to move towards a holistic perspective, I am with those who also see the spiritual as needing to be reintegrated as well. The research bears this out.

Up to now, we have emphasized the mental and physical capacities available to you for making marked improvement to mental health, here and now. What cannot be described or achieved through those avenues may be accessed through the spiritual. Though it is nuanced, harder to define and therefore harder to utilize, I find that research and clinical observation indicate that it is worthy of your time and attention. Our posture in approaching all of these resources matters. Attentional bias is the term for the way the brain prioritizes selecting certain information for processing (MacLeod et al., 2023). We find what we are looking for. If we are looking for evidence that God is not there, or that the spiritual does not exist, I'm sure you will find evidence to convince yourself of that argument. Similarly, if you look for evidence of a soul, you will find it. As we have endeavored to approach each resource with mindful intention, I invite you to approach soul and its role in mental wellness with renewed openness and attention.

As there are parts of the human experience that seem to be unthinkable, we find in the human design an ability to exist within experiences that defy explanation. Most specifically, I refer to the excruciating, the grotesque, and the wrong that cannot be explained away and will not end up okay. If there is a part of us that is beyond what can be seen and understood that connects to something larger than ourselves, then we possess an untouchable quality and unshakable meaning that can be of particular relief to those for whom life has included unanswerable suffering. As Otto Rank said, "The immortal soul, whether fact or fiction, gives comfort" (Pandya, 2011). As determining the fact or fiction of the soul is far beyond the scope of this work, our focus for this resource remains where it can and will provide us comfort.

In Defense of Soul in Mental Health

At times, some in the field of psychology are quick to find a "reasonable" explanation for what seems spiritual or otherworldly. In fields of science, those of the opinion that the spiritual does not exist are termed "materialist." This is not a small portion of the world of scientists. The materialist view "requires all events to have a material cause, which means a cause governed by the physical forces of nature" (Beauregard and O'Leary, 2007). The nonmaterialist view, on the other hand, retains openness to the forces outside of physical nature to exist, to have potential impact, and to produce phenomena observable in the physical world. Both, though for different reasons, verify the benefit of religious or spiritual experiences on mental health. At this point, the valid use of spirituality within mental health is broadly acknowledged (Verghese, 2008).

With most ameliorating, beneficial results in psychological research, we seem to give positive assumptions with positive results except when it comes to the spiritual. As most research points to the need for further research, evidence of benefit is reason enough to promote a practice even while the mechanism is unclear. In other words, there is a readiness and a comfort to keep moving forward with an intervention that has positive results even if we don't fully understand how it works.

When it comes to the spiritual, that default or positive assumption doesn't always exist. The documented and verifiable data of the benefits of spiritual engagement, like any other beneficial practices or intervention in psychology, merits credence and application. Spirituality in mental health is not serving as a silver bullet, but it does provide the needed balance to a thorough approach to whole-person mental wellness (Verghese, 2008).

THE SCIENCE OF SOUL

In various forms of spiritual practice, research has tracked positive benefits in the brain and body (Lucchetti et al., 2021). There are desirable, tangible effects worth pursuing. There is something different about these practices in that the benefits are not simply due to the practice itself, but the additional component of drawing from a source distinct from the brain or body. **Soul provides the means to both improve mental wellness within the brain and body and to seek wellness beyond mental and physical limits.** As the resource of soul is distinct from other resources, our approach in considering its effectiveness is similarly nuanced. As a key component is belief, the first point will look at some neuroscience surrounding the soul and ideas of consciousness. By looking at the shadow, we may get some useful idea of the form and its function for mental wellness. Then, a brief exploration of research demonstrating the benefits of spirituality will follow. Before getting into the practices, there will be a focus on how the integration of the soul with the brain and body is necessary and practical.

Indications of Soul from Neuroscience

To look to the soul is to look beyond the natural limits of the brain and body, and so it is to look beyond the typical limits of science. Neuroscience defending the soul relies on observations of the physical in response to the unobservable. One fascinating approach to this is the research of people with near-death experiences (NDEs). As this is a relatively new-on-the-scene area of study due to medical developments that enable people to be resuscitated, the terminology and defining of relevant terms are still being agreed upon. Some call them "recalled experiences of death" or "authentic NDEs" (Parnia et al., 2022). For our discussion, we will use the term NDE.

Now, the context of these NDEs is not an adrenaline sport or narrow escape of some misfortune. In the scientific research of NDEs, the individual being studied must have experienced and have documented "clinical death," in which the brain and body show no activity (Beauregard & O'Leary, 2007). As you can imagine, such examples are rare and even more difficult to report. When it is documented, the data is compelling.

Most of these events are documented in medical settings such as life-saving procedures. Individuals with NDEs report after the fact that during the time when they were in reality "clinically dead," they were able to observe parts of medical procedures, overhear conversation, and have multisensory experiences all while the brain was registering "no activity." What is exceptionally odd about these reports is the accuracy of their accounts. Some report the conversations happening in the operating room, the types of tools used during the surgery, or where their personal belongings were placed while they were under (Beauregard & O'Leary, 2007).

Within the data, there is evidence of a part of the self not fully explained by and limited to the brain and body. The indication is that the consciousness of self – the soul – can be present when clinical criteria of death is met. Often, those who have had a NDE convey the experience as "spiritual" or transformative. The implication here is that an element of spiritual practices function in part in dependence on and conjunction with the brain, and yet also with an element of independence from it (Beauregard & O'Leary, 2007).

Though NDEs are not a common human experience, the growing body of literature reports similar experiences of a revelatory and subsequently transformational nature (Parnia et al., 2022). It is odd that the report back of what is experienced when in a state of "clinical death" has numerous accurate details and stranger still that it all would result in improvement to the mental well-being of the person after resuscitation. The objective isn't to seek out NDEs, but to acknowledge the verifiable neuroscience confirming what you may suspect: that there is more to you than meets the eye, more to you than your brain and body. What's more, there is a flourishing of mental wellness that comes with connecting to the soul, to experiences aligned with the spiritual part of our holistic person.

Similar but distinct from NDEs, there are records of people experiencing a paradoxical form of consciousness that their terminal illness or vegetative state would deem impossible (Parnia et al., 2022). When consciousness seems gone, and when the broken body ceases to respond, an element remains that can later affirm that an awareness and sense of self remains. When observable data indicates lack of physical sensation or correlated levels of decreased brain activity, a consciousness or form of being beyond observable data exists. This can all be debated. However, what we are interested in with the mental health resource of the soul is the transformational benefits that seem to be connected with that transcendental belief or experience beyond the confines of just the brain and body.

The resource of the soul certainly functions within your brain and body; we are holistic beings. However, it also is not wholly limited to the physical and mental. For those with certain physical or mental impairments, this is good news. For those without the obvious impairments, it is also needed and good news. There is a resource that you can draw from beyond physical limits or mental hardships, an available experience of connection that brings desired change, healing, and soothing.

Benefits of Intrinsic Spirituality

It may be difficult to demonstrate the mechanisms of how people glean from spiritual practices, especially the elements that may lie beyond observable brain activity. However, we can observe the results for those who pursue belief or practice connection with spirituality. These results are another shadow of sorts, giving shape to the shapeless. The results are clear: mental health improves with engaging the soul. Our pursuit is not proof of the improvable but rather the posturing toward belief that has benefited humans from the beginning of time.

In a Gallup report from 2022, a strong correlation appears between religious/spiritual engagement and general well-being. Americans who describe themselves as "very religious" are reportedly happier and healthier (Newport, 2022). In 2012 a systematic review was done of research from peer-reviewed studies between 1872 and 2010 on the effects of religion/spirituality on mental and physical health. That's over a century's worth of data synthesized to gain a generalized picture. The study demonstrated that religion/spirituality had positive correlations with hope, meaning and purpose, desired emotions, and especially coping with internal or external adversity. It was summarized that though the resource of soul "is not a panacea, on the balance, it is generally associated with greater well-being, improved coping with stress, and better mental health" (Koenig, 2012).

There are different potential reasons for this improvement, some of which are the social community that can come with religious involvement, the benefits of belonging to a group with a belief beyond the self, and regular practices of care for others. These characteristics are considered "extrinsic faith," a spirituality that has to do with identifying with a religious group or external practices. And although there is clear, supported evidence of the benefit of such involvement (Shattuck & Muehlenbein, 2020), the evidence equally supports use of "intrinsic" faith or spirituality.

"Intrinsic faith" has to do with the internal experience of a person. The neuroscience of the soul examines, among other things, events called "religious, spiritual, mystical experiences," or RSMEs. In studies examining the beneficial aspects of such experiences, it has been found that the operating factor is "intrinsic faith." In other words, the agent of change is the authentic, personal experience of engaging the part of us not totally described by brain or by body in a posture of expanding beyond the self (Beauregard and O'Leary, 2007). As our focus is the most available, most accessible aspect of each resource, our focus on soul will be the reality and pursuit of "intrinsic" spiritual practice.

The Practice of Spirituality and Soul

Albert Einstein spoke to the necessity for a central spirituality:

> When you examine the lives of the most influential people who have ever walked among us, you discover one thread that winds through them all.

> They have been aligned first with their spiritual nature and only then with their physical selves. (Francini, 2012)

His scientific observation noticed that those who attained more optimal functioning lived with an orientation between themselves and the transcendental. Humans are at their best when guided in part by spiritual practice.

The medical field at large is continuing the trend toward reunifying the brain-body-soul components in more holistic approaches to disease, wellness, and all that's in between. Mental health therapies, psychology, and psychiatry are similarly responding to the documented efficacy of treating the whole person. Interventions for mental health that prioritize the spiritual are on the rise. In a broad review of randomized controlled trials testing effectiveness of mental health approaches targeting mind, body, and spirit, an incredible 83% were found to yield positive results. And equally as impressive, none of the interventions revealed any negative result or adverse side effects – none (Lee et al., 2018). We often willingly attempt and continue with treatments with numbers far less compelling than these. Besides the potentially polarizing nature in the various values of spirituality, I think the reason why many fail to attempt spiritual practices for mental health is that there isn't a clear, practical path forward.

The gap between soul and mind can be tapered with concepts of ethics or morality, the overlap of where belief influences values and then practice. Belief in the beyond informs a positive ethic that pursues good and truth, fosters compassion, and practices communally in trust of a higher Truth (Junaidi et al., 2022). As these demonstrate positive effects for mental wellness (Lucchetti et al., 2021), it is worth reiterating that the catalyst is the belief of the supernatural, of the self beyond the physical, and not simply a belief in the efficacy of the practice. The spiritual roots that hold fast Virtue, Morality, and Justice are the same roots providing nourishment for mental well-being, enabling a healing that can spring forth amidst contrary situations and limits of person.

Even as we acknowledge aspects of the soul that may not be totally understood or captured within data, our approach to it as a resource is meant to be decidedly practical and easy to access. Indeed, spiritual practices can provide a natural ground upon which we can build effective interventions (Plante, 2009). A simple approach to integrate the soul in the brain-body-soul triad is to create practical overlaps between spiritual practice with mental health (Junaidi et al., 2022). We can do this by pairing long-lived spiritual traditions with proven practices of mental health. Such spiritual traditions may include belief, conviction of the immortal, an awareness of something bigger than ourselves, or faith in Truth and Goodness. Established practices of mental health could be mindfulness meditation, breath work, thought selection, and so on. Some common overlap between the two are found in practices such as prayer, forgiveness, gratitude, giving, and the like. In many ways it's an instinctive partnership that finds application in ordinary, everyday life.

SOUL IN PRACTICE

The role of spirituality in mental wellness is widely accepted. The presence of the soul is reflected in neuroscience and drawn upon practically in psychotherapy. It rests with each of us to proceed as we are willing. **We practice soul by pairing traditions of belief with practical mental health interventions.** Whether consideration of spirituality is new territory for you or if the roots of faith for you run deep, optimal application of the resource of soul lies in ongoing practice.

> Many people in present-day societies long to develop their spiritual side, but they wonder whether it really exists . . . Their spiritual side does indeed exist. But like any faculty, it must be allowed to develop if they would like to see their lives transformed. (Beauregard and O'Leary, 2007)

Development of the soul component of the brain-body-soul triad comes with simple, consistent engagement. The following practices are meant as a clear path in that direction.

Meditation Practice – Meditation Pairing Breath and Belief

On the firm ground of mindfulness, the meditation will contemplate the limits of the brain and body. Meditations like these, incorporating brain, body, and spirit, demonstrate unique benefits in comparison to meditation of the strictly brain-body variety (Joshi et al., 2022). Just as individually there is an aspect of each person that exists distinct from the confines of the brain and body, it is useful to consider the broader scope, an environment beyond the physical and mental limits in which we live and move. The basic premise of this meditation is meant to be available for anyone at any point of belief by pairing meditation with an open consideration of the Good and the True that exists beyond our limits. Go to kristaagler.com/book/keepinmind to listen to the provided audio or follow the accompanying prompts for this guided meditation pairing breath and belief.

Reflection Practice – A Perspective Pairing Mindfulness and Hope

Mindfulness refers to a mindset that is cultivated to be in the present moment, paying attention, and doing so without judgment. The ongoing conscious awareness of the self in a manner that is open, alert, and kind results in sweeping mental health benefits (Zhang et al., 2021). "Hope" may be viewed from a variety of perspectives. On the one hand, the overtly religious definition of hope may include faith as well as the specific object of faith. On the other hand, the psychological perspective sees hope as a cognitive effort with effects on both emotions and actions, specifically naming the mechanisms of envisioning a desired good and committing to moving that direction (Corn et al., 2020). For the practice at hand, it will be conceptualized somewhere in between. Hope is belief in and movement toward the unseen good. It may be specific, as in hoping for a specific medical-test result or election outcome. It may be more broad, like the desire for and belief that what is wrong could be made right.

For the reflection practice, respond to the prompts in Table 13.1 regarding your current experience of belief and spirituality. Approach each question with a focus on the present moment, this very moment. Also, try to do so without judging your responses as good or bad; simply acknowledge them as noticed details of your current state. Tethered to both mindfulness and hope, we can encourage a mindset that draws from the source of soul in an accessible, therapeutic way.

Conscious Practice – Pairing Prayer and Acceptance

When I envision prayer, one image that comes to mind is my friend's mother who, in profound grief, repeatedly returned to her prayer rug. In visits for tea, I witnessed the tearful kneeling, facing east. My friend told of finding her mother finally asleep after unending prayer on the thinning fabric that had become her place of solace. Prayer has been a pillar across religions, and at present most people pray regularly (Froese & Jones, 2021). Prayer, for all of human history, has been a shared place of comfort when no tangible lifelines appear.

Acceptance is a fitting companion for prayer. It is a conscious posture of acknowledging present thoughts, emotions, situations, and so forth with a mind to cease changing the unchangeable. There are formal applications for acceptance in mental health therapy that result in decreased symptoms and improved quality of life (Rahnama Zadeh et al., 2022). In a practice of prayer, acceptance is not a stance of resignation; it's a posture of presentation, open to surrender and receptivity. The following prayer practice incorporates acceptance, lends itself to repetition, and supports mental wellness.

Come to a place of physical stillness. Sit comfortably on a chair, lay supine on the firm ground, or stand in easy balance. With open hands, mentally extend the statement, "Here I am." In offering an external communication, it is a statement acknowledging a higher power. It is a statement of presence and availability. It is a statement of receptivity as well as acceptance. It is prayer. The prayer offers the outgoing message, reaching past limits of the brain and body. It provides an opportunity to posture toward receiving with that which is beyond limits of brain logic or body response.

Perhaps morning and night, perhaps at a few timed intervals throughout the day, perhaps as needed, take a momentary pause to breathe mindfully, still your posture, and mentally pray "Here I am."

Table 13.1 *A Perspective of Mindfulness and Hope*

Prompt	Response
What is your current relationship to belief and spirituality?	
What is your current interest in or desire for belief or faith?	
Notice the presence of both belief and doubt, observing them equally. What do you notice?	
What unseen good do you want to see materialize? Be specific and general. Think short term and long term.	
What might it be like to attempt more or any belief in the possibility of the unseen good?	
What might it look like to believe and move toward the unseen good?	

Lifestyle Practice – Holistic Mental Health Pairing Mindset and Faith

Through the exploration of these many resources, the goal has been to find ways to incorporate them into regular life so that drawing from them and using them becomes second nature. Though formal practices or habits are part of the aim, cultivating a mindset is ideal. We must begin with some conscious intention and regular use until newly formed neural pathways become well-established and self-sustaining.

The resource of soul is innate in each person, boasting positive effect in practice and bringing completion to the brain-body-soul holism within which the human system best functions. Imagining we each had a bank set aside specifically for investing in the spiritual arena, we would do well to make regular contributions. That is the task before us.

There is a text in my faith tradition that says of us: "They should seek God, and perhaps feel their way toward him and find him. Yet he is actually not far from each one of us" (English Standard Version Bible, 2001, Acts 17:27). The deeper meaning of the Greek word from which the phrase "feel their way toward" comes is to "mentally seek after tokens of a person or thing." So, one way we invest in that resource bank is to set an attentional bias with a mind to seek after tokens or evidence of the soul. With an openness to the potential of a consciousness not limited to our brain and body, we may discover with our senses such tokens. With a leaning toward the existence of something other, toward hope and the unseen good, toward acceptance and prayer, we similarly collect findings from which our mental and physical self connects to something beyond. The stance is not conjuring sentimentality; it is sifting methodically and energetically through the sand for tangible coins of evidence. Simply put: If you were to look at your life, past and present, what is the evidence of soul that you find? And could you give mental attention to collecting that evidence in conjunction with your efforts for mental wellness?

IN SUMMARY

"When Breath Becomes Air" is the breathtaking and gritty memoir of neurosurgeon Paul Kalanithi and his journey on two tandem paths: completing residency and navigating his cancer diagnosis, which led to his early death. His account of his life is a window into a unique perspective acutely zeroed in on both the physical wonder of the human brain and the distinctive meaning within human consciousness. Of his hallowed role in performing patients' surgeries as well as attending to their values and personhood, he said, "The call to protect life – and not merely life but another's identity; it is perhaps not too much to say another's soul – was obvious in its sacredness" (2016). His story demonstrates not only the human need to see both the physical and the spiritual, but also the surprisingly fitting and natural place they have together.

Humans are host to a consciousness that has some distinction from limits of the brain and body. Relating to this spiritual part of ourselves catalyzes mental wellness. With simple, intrinsic practices of belief, humans have the ability to integrate soul in the brain-body-soul triad effectively. Regardless of your history or previous exposure to spirituality, there is unseen Good that can be sought, collected, and internalized. Soul, for all that is unexplained, is a demonstratively practical part of the pursuit of mental wellness.

REFERENCES

Beauregard, M., & O'Leary, D. (2007). *The spiritual brain: A neuroscientist's case for the existence of the soul.* HarperOne.

Corn, B. W., Feldman, D. B., & Wexler, I. (2020). The science of hope. *The Lancet Oncology, 21*(9), e452–e459.

English Standard Version Bible. (2001). Acts 17:27. *Crossway.*

Froese, P., & Jones, R. (2021). The sociology of prayer: Dimensions and mechanisms. *Social Sciences, 10*(1), 15.

Jones, J.M. (2022, June 17). Belief in God in U.S. dips to 81%, a new low. *Gallup.*

Joshi, S. P., Wong, A. K. I., Brucker, A., Ardito, T. A., Chow, S. C., Vaishnavi, S., & Lee, P. J. (2022). Efficacy of transcendental meditation to reduce stress among health care workers: A randomized clinical trial. *JAMA Network Open, 5*(9), Article e2231917

Junaidi, J., Anriani, H.B., Sari, H., Hamka, H. (2022). Investigating the relationship between moral and ethical: Does extrinsic and intrinsic religiosity improve people's mental health? *FWU Journal of Social Science, 16*(3), 52–67

Kalanithi, P. (2016). *When breath becomes air.* (1st ed.). Random House.

Koenig, H.G. (2012, December 16). Religion, spirituality, and health: The research and clinical implications. *ISRN Psychiatry.*

Lee, M. Y., Wang, X., Liu, C., Raheim, S., & Tebb, S. (2018). Outcome literature review of integrative body–mind–spirit practices for mental health conditions. *Social Work Research, 42*(3), 251–266.

Leibowitz, K. A., Hardebeck, E. J., Goyer, J. P., & Crum, A. J. (2019). The role of patient beliefs in open-label placebo effects. *Health Psychology, 38*(7), 613.

Lucchetti, G., Koenig, H. G., & Lucchetti, A. L. G. (2021). Spirituality, religiousness, and mental health: A review of the current scientific evidence. *World Journal of Clinical Cases, 9*(26), 7620.

Luccio, R. (2013). Psychologia–the birth of a new scientific context. *Review of Psychology, 20*(1–2), 5–14.

MacLeod, C. (2023). The attention bias modification approach to anxiety: Origins, limitations, and opportunities. *American Journal of Psychiatry, 180*(5), 328–330.

Merriam-Webster. (n.d.). Soul. In *Merriam-Webster.com* dictionary. Retrieved January 21, 2024, from https://www.merriam-webster.com/dictionary/soul

Newport, F. (2022, February 4). Religion and well-being in the U.S.: Update. *Gallup.*

Pandya, S. K. (2011). Understanding brain, mind and soul: Contributions from neurology and neurosurgery. *Mens Sana Monographs, 9*(1), 129–49.

Parnia, S., Post, S. G., Lee, M. T., Lyubomirsky, S., Aufderheide, T. P., Deakin, C. D., Greyson, B., Long, J., Gonzales, A. M., Huppert, E. L., Dickinson, A., Mayer, S., Locicero, B., Levin, J., Bossis, A., Worthington, E., Fenwick, P., & Shirazi, T. K. (2022). Guidelines and standards for the study of death and recalled experiences of death—a multidisciplinary consensus statement and proposed future directions. *Annals of the New York Academy of Sciences, 1511*(1), 5–21.

Plante, T. G. (2009). *Spiritual practices in psychotherapy: Thirteen tools for enhancing psychological health.* American Psychological Association.

Rahnama Zadeh, M., Ashayerih, H., Ranjbaripour, T., Kakavand, A., & Meschi, F. (2022). The effectiveness of acceptance and commitment therapy on depression, alexithymia and hypertension in patients with coronary heart disease. *International Clinical Neuroscience Journal, 9*(1).

Shattuck, E. C., & Muehlenbein, M. P. (2020). Religiosity/spirituality and physiological markers of health. *Journal of religion and health, 59*(2), 1035–1054.

Southwick, S. M., Lowthert, B. T., Graber, A. V. (2016). Logotherapy and existential analysis: Proceedings of the Viktor Frankl Institute Vienna. In *Relevance and application of logotherapy to enhance resilience to stress and trauma* (Vol. 1, pp. 131–149). Springer.

Verghese, A. (2008). Spirituality and mental health. *Indian Journal of Psychiatry, 50*(4), 233–237.

Zhang, D., Lee, E. K., Mak, E. C., Ho, C. Y., & Wong, S. Y. (2021). Mindfulness-based interventions: an overall review. *British Medical Bulletin, 138*(1), 41–57.

Chapter 14

Contribution: A Resource of Paradoxical Happiness

Sophie's demeanor had a certain grace, even though she had been yellowed by the years: skin not quite vibrant, teeth uniformly stained, and hair brassy gray. Her features were lovely, but her brow seemed perpetually furrowed in suspicion of people. She went to therapy for the first time in her later years, nearing retirement. She was left by her husband, who she should have left long before, as she tells it. After decades, her now ex-husband had found a way to get her name off some legal documents that would have required him to split a portion of his inheritance with her. In the meantime, Sophie had survived the violent marriage and made a life out of compliance, thinking it would one day secure her safety, and yet here she was, old and with next to nothing. For the entirety of her life, she had been abused – by her dad beginning at the age of six, by a teacher throughout her high school years, and then by a boyfriend who would become her husband for 30 years. She had been violated, shamed, wounded.

She had no children, and lived now in an apartment she could cover with her job answering phones for a telecommunications company. Since her husband left her, her schedule was now vacant, released from his control. She seemed to stare at the time, almost frozen with freedom. Some time into her trauma treatment, she responded to an internal suspicion that she had untapped "mother love" within her. She began volunteering at the local NICU (neonatal intensive care unit) holding premature babies. She increased her hours at the NICU until she was volunteering the equivalent of a part-time job in addition to her essential full-time one.

She spoke of the work: "They need the regulation. The babies. Breathing and skin contact. Some of their parents can't be there all the time. I have

DOI: 10.4324/9781003521945-18

breath and I have skin, and I always wanted to have babies to hold. And maybe they're regulating me. Don't know if I ever had that."

As she continued her trauma treatment, she gingerly unpacked in daylight the stories that were held in shadowed silence for too long. She kept volunteering at the NICU, and over time, she decreased the frequency of appointments. Every other week. Monthly. Until one day she stopped all of it: Therapy. Volunteering. Her job.

Her eyes would twinkle as she told the few people in her life she thought would care. "I've quit my job. I'm moving to Southern Asia to help an organization that works with mothers giving birth to premature babies. I leave in two weeks with a one way ticket."

She came back for a brief stint to relinquish her apartment and her remaining belongings before returning to her new home. She was radiant and well, actually looking younger and healthier than years before; her face softer and rosy. She would say that she had a new life and that a number of things were responsible for that. At the top of the list, it was finding there was a need for her to give of herself, and the experience of being transformed by contributing. Betting all she had, she left what she knew and gave herself to a full life some will never experience.

THE NATURE OF CONTRIBUTION

We each have had our share of suffering, some more than a fair share. Mental distress has a way of draining resources of all kinds. The nature of life has demands: labor, responsibility, survival, and effort, at the very least. The idea of "giving back" when you're already down may seem unreasonable. Yet clients from my clinical experience come to mind and, perhaps like you, even after the most severe trauma and even in some of the most precarious days of the recovery journey, they were already postured to give back, to give to others. It's as if through the hardship that a well of compassion and an ability to understand the need in others materializes. There is research that speaks to the experience, for indeed, increased suffering produces increased compassion and a tendency to act to alleviate the suffering of others (Lim & DeSteno, 2016). For many, it is nature to see and meet other people's needs.

For others, it's possible that loss, trauma, and mental health struggle can create a narrative believing that there is absolutely nothing left – nothing to give. For those of you that feel this way, perhaps a time in the future will come when you feel you have something to contribute, though I suspect that even now you possess merit, as you are, that could do good for another. Perhaps after all you've been through, you've latched onto the message that giving of yourself was something you should stop doing.

The message is flawed. Perhaps you need proper limits in giving of yourself, but to stop all contribution is to limit healing and happiness. In using the resource of contribution, the emphasis is on an internal locus of control, on giving on purpose. With contribution, no one is forcing you, yet in freely giving, we set off a mental chain of events that makes for improved well-being.

So the goal becomes redirecting attention from the lack that would be a barrier to contributing and focusing instead on the, perhaps, small amount each has to give. The skill of shifting perspective comes into play in a powerful way here. Often what prevents us from giving, taking part, or contributing are the very real aspects of where we are without. The deficit can tell a story of limit, of uselessness. By reframing slightly, we soon discover there is almost always something we have that we can spare that meets someone else's need. Perhaps because we know we can't do more, we too quickly forfeit the opportunity to contribute. With contribution and mental health, a little may be enough.

Contribution is the "giving or supplying of something that plays a significant part in making something happen" (Merriam-Webster, n.d.). It's an exertion that compounds and diversifies the investment, impacting recipient and benefactor alike. It is effort that initiates surplus rather than deficit. Contribution is like kinetic energy in you, the motion of outpouring creates new internal reserves. **Contribution is the resource of the ability to give that is essential to the full experience of mental wellness**.

Essential to the resource of contribution is that you are the only one who can initiate it. Contribution, and how it works in the brain and body, is not meant to be done under the pressure of others (Collett & Morrissey, 2007). It is not the result of guilt or of being deceived. It is a product of choice, an effort of ourselves for the voluntary betterment of another. It's not just a random act of kindness; it's an intentional mechanism within the brain. Contribution is work or effort given in generosity, aware of the cost, with the reliable outcome of our own good.

The human system responds to a variety of interactions with contribution. Simply witnessing acts of kindness induces more pleasant emotions. Interactions of caring for another enhance the effect, increasing resilience and reducing the negative effects of chronic stress (Fryburg, 2022). By cultivating some of the characteristics associated with contribution such as kindness, generosity, love, and the like not only improve mental health, but offset the experience of suffering (Niemiec, 2023). Though the opportunities for contribution are as numerous as there are people, by focusing simply on a couple arenas, we begin to shape practical steps to make it part of life, and part of ongoing mental health care.

The Contribution in Work

Using the resource of contribution may require some added output. Maybe not. It may simply require refocusing your attention on ways you are already working at cost to yourself for the good of another. We may take for granted the effort we put into the "daily grind," which may be a significant source of contribution we overlook due to its ordinariness. Perhaps the place for you to begin consideration of this resource is where you are already exerting effort and mentally connecting it to ways that your work provides for others, even if it also provides for you. Whether it supports your family, provides a needed or desirable service for others, cares for dependents, or is necessary for functioning of society at large, contribution as a resource takes care to consider what your exertion brings, large or small.

Work can impact the basic functioning of the world while also serving to boost mental health. "Working represents a core aspect of human life, optimally providing a means of sustainability, social connection and contribution, self-determination, and a source of meaning" (Blustein et al., 2023). To be clear, work could be a paid position or unpaid. Work is wherever we exert ourselves toward a useful end. As work meets practical needs and is often accomplished in conjunction with others, it serves multiple aspects of our brain-body system. Even more, the effect of accomplishment on a person and the pride of being a part of something is no small matter. In fact, research indicates that a lack of work has a negative impact on physical and mental health (Waddell & Burton, 2006). In your work, where your effort costs you and benefits another, you are contributing. In really noticing and honoring the contribution you are already engaged in, you access the brain-level shift toward happiness that comes with it.

The Contribution in Generosity

The full benefit of contribution is experienced not only as work, but also as generosity. One definition of generosity is "the virtue of giving good things to others freely and abundantly. What exactly generosity gives can be various things: money, possessions, time, attention, aid, encouragement, emotional availability, and more" (Allen, 2018). If generosity is the virtue, then contribution is the act.

Neurologically speaking, humans have the capacity for both selfish behaviors and for generous behaviors. Generosity, by its nature, is costly because it transfers some resource from yourself (time, energy) to the account of another (Park et al., 2017). Even so, we find extensive biological and developmental roots demonstrating the centrality of generosity in human functioning. Even more than that, studies on humans consistently find that freely engaging in the costly work of generosity for others results in better overall health and reduced psychological distress (Allen, 2018). There is a neural transaction that alters the equation. That which we suspect will rob us actually brings back dividends of mental health relief and ushers the brain into its instinctive capacity for happiness.

Contribution functions directly in increasing positive emotions. The change happens through "altruistic attitudes," volunteering, and even casual efforts to help. Pause here and notice that simply an "altruistic attitude" can bring psychological benefits. It should not be overlooked that even before any action or cost occurs, the mindset of wanting to give can have an impact on emotional state. It's available to anyone, even when we find ourselves with very real limitations of exerting ourselves for others. So, "having a 'generous spirit', even when it may be difficult to act on that spirit, can help maintain positive emotions" (Allen, 2018). The resource is available to all.

The research on the human brain and its functioning indicates that all people have the capacity for generosity, from intention to action. It also shows that often, people have a tendency to neglect use of this capacity, and then forego the support that accompanies it. There seems to be a cultural tendency to function from the belief that happiness comes by prioritizing ourselves, but research indicates that contributing and emphasizing others actually generates happiness (Allen, 2018).

When I think about my clients who have lost the most, those who have suffered the most, every single one of them consciously, deliberately gives of themselves, as if their life depends on it in some instances. And perhaps it does. Out of and in spite of great suffering remains the human capacity to play a significantly needed part. Then, out of and maybe because of your contribution, you participate in the collective onset of mental wellness.

THE SCIENCE OF CONTRIBUTION

While allowing us to be a needed part of someone else's need fulfillment, contributing brings about deeper healing and exponential vibrancy to ourselves. It is the necessary result of our brains' natural function and wiring. **Contribution provides means to encourage brain-based well-being for ourselves, activated by effort for others.**

Hardwired for Contribution

As psychologists and neurologists continue to study the generosity of humans, the trajectory is clear: our brains are more positively activated by giving than receiving (Karajagi, 2014). When we act in a way that benefits others, even at our own cost, neural circuits awaken and trigger reward systems similar to when we eat really good food or have sex. "Humans are born with the biological hardware required for generosity. In particular, we have brain circuits and hormone systems in place and at the ready that help us help others – and make us feel good while doing so" (Allen, 2018).

Providing something that benefits others is key in contribution. The neural circuitry shifts depending on whether an action is "for me" or "for others" (Palermo, 2023). At a brain level, we assess the pros and cons of each decision we make. Our brain interprets both decisions that benefit ourselves and decisions that benefit others in a "common currency" so that we have the opportunity to choose when to act in our own interest and when to act to help others. It's not always that simple, but those are the basic two directions, and both are necessary at times. What is key here is that the domino effect of happiness is initiated when we act for the benefit of others. Really think about this: your and my brain function in a way that happiness is more reliably secured by giving to others than doing for ourselves.

A reminder here that the giving has to be by free choice and consciously done. Limits need to be considered for sustainability and intentionality. Giving in a way that is self-determined, mindful, and presently engaged ensures that you are doing it well.

In a study done on helping, simply agreeing to help brought a rise in mood, though the act of helping brought the most significant positive shift. Fascinatingly, those in the study who were directed to do something for themselves reported no emotional benefit. Defying expectation, the group that received the most direct advantage did not experience the ultimately desired outcome of more well-being. Giving money to others, no matter the level of disposable income, brought about a noticeable increase in happiness, while there was no correlation with spending money on oneself and a real experience of happiness. Studies revealed that even small amounts of money that were intentionally directed to another brought noticeable and sustainable happiness. Interestingly, most subjects recorded in these studies assumed that spending on oneself would make them happier, which is reflective of the general population (Allen, 2018).

Our brains are wired to find well-being in giving, yet messages of self-serving are abound. As humans, we have a belief that we will be happier the more we obtain for ourselves, and yet we house wiring that charges with happiness when contributing to others. We are wired, from a basic brain level, to be happier and healthier when contributing to others within our limits.

Neuroscience of Contribution and Happiness

A key part of the brain involved with generosity components of contribution is the temporoparietal junction (TPJ). The word "junction" is an apt description because its location is a connecting point between a number of brain regions, and even more so because it orchestrates the various information pathways crossing between regions. Think of a train junction, or a train station that is a central point for many different tracks. The TPJ is an intersection coordinating information from different "destinations." From both interoceptive and exteroceptive senses, from visual and auditory data, from the limbic system (pain, pleasure, and rage) as well as the sensorimotor functions, these trains are coming in and out, dropping off and picking up passengers. The junction handles all of this with regulation and optimization. And this junction, this TPJ, is integral in generosity (Park et al., 2017).

The TPJ is associated with discerning between the self and other people. It also is instrumental in the specific distinction between our own pain and the pain of others. Understandably, it is a region of the brain associated with empathy (Stevens & Taber, 2021). It's not hard to detect how this region comes into play with contribution. There is a brain-based ability to see the other as other, to see their hardship, and to weigh the cost of taking on some discomfort, inconvenience, or even pain in order to alleviate the pain of another.

As the TPJ serves as a major modulator of various brain activity, one of its responsibilities is the monitoring of happiness. It does not register happiness in a "get more, be happier" program. It is a "generous-behavior-dependent" mechanism. It activates "trains" that increase happiness as we make generous decisions. Uniquely, "the TPJ showed increased activity especially when participants chose to forgo their own rewards in favour of rewards for others" (Park et al., 2017).

The TPJ, this grand-central station of regulation that sets happiness in motion, lights up most when we sacrifice for the benefit of others. It's a mental experience of empathy that registers more with cognition than with emotion; it is a deliberate calculation (Stevens & Taber, 2021). Although it's part of our basic neurological functioning, there is a strong social construction working against it. The belief is prevalent that happiness will come from what we acquire, or at least with what works for us. The TPJ tells a different story: happiness comes with the cost we consciously and willingly spend for others.

The Happy Cost in Contribution

Though the presence of cost inherent to contribution may seem initially off putting, it becomes hopeful in that it can make good use of the mental and emotional costs of living. The cost-happiness relationship within contribution makes for a major shift in narrative. That which costs you may not ultimately be for your detriment. It may be the making of a life experienced with pleasure and satisfaction. The functional duality within the human brain opens a door to more well-being and happiness beyond a closed equation of "more is more, better is better." If cost is part of the equation of happiness, then some of what seems an expense could actually be investment. Cost is not an obstacle to happiness.

For many trauma survivors, in my clinical observation, finding ways to "give back" as a result of the trauma can be pivotal in recovery. Research following those who survive trauma depicts a phenomenon termed "posttraumatic growth," which is "the transformative positive change that can come about as a result of the struggle with highly challenging life crises" (Tedeschi & Calhoun, 2004). One manifestation of posttraumatic growth is "sensemaking," or reorienting after a trauma by reclaiming purpose (Maitlis, 2020). Finding ways to improve the lives of others directly because of the trauma is profound sensemaking. The cost that represents their suffering is remade into contribution, providing something significantly needed for others.

There are some specifics of how the generosity of contribution ideally works. Interpersonal acts of giving are more beneficial than using a go-between as there are social and sensory aspects to experiencing kindness in person by both the giver and the recipient (Nelson et al., 2016). People are happiest when they get to engage in contribution that has a social component, that is clear to how their effort/gift has made a difference, and that contribution is their free choice. The brain doesn't want to be generous at a distance; it doesn't want to outsource the process, but to be directly involved.

By committing to be generous (intention) we are then more generous (by will), and experience the resulting happiness and well-being at a neural level (Park et al., 2017). When we intentionally override egocentric tendencies and freely choose to sacrificially give to others, the brain responds positively with happiness, as if it's what it is meant to do. There seems to be a symbiotic nature rather than a transactional one when it comes to contribution.

CONTRIBUTION IN PRACTICE

More than a onetime donation or an occasional act of kindness to pay forward, our aim is cultivating a way of being. Just as a breathing practice will eventually lead to healthier breath at all times, practices of contribution direct us toward generous living. There is no reason to make the practice infrequent. With proper limits and pacing, incorporating regular practices of contribution are not likely to cause deficit or drain. The research speaks to the contrary; regularly taking part in mindful giving for the good of another not only serves the community, but your brain-body system as well. Contribution is not a romanticized ideal but an effective intervention and preventative measure. **We practice contribution through purposefully giving to others, while aware of the cost, in pursuit of a lifestyle of generosity.**

Meditation Practice – A Guided Meditation for a Mindset of Generosity

Simply cultivating a mindset of altruism, even before action is taken, has a positive effect on mental health. Meditation with specific visualizations can help create some neural connections preparing you for contribution. Go to kristaagler.com/book/keepinmind to listen to the provided audio or follow the accompanying prompts for this guided meditation for a mindset of generosity.

Reflection Practice – Mindfully Meeting Needs with Enough

Enough doesn't mean all you could want or all that you may have in the future. Enough is a sufficient portion for the moment. An imbalance of attention on the lack will drown out the sufficiency in enough. We discover our capacity for contribution by reflecting on where we have enough, today. Contributing takes two parts: acknowledging what you have to give and finding a place to give it. At times, it's sufficient to see what you have to give and generally make it available: Donating clothes. Providing canned goods and toiletries for a local shelter. Other times, we have to go a step further and look with awareness to pinpoint where there is need. It may help to begin with those closest to you and even acquaintances with whom you have regular contact. We won't have to look far, and we don't have to look hard. The world over is saturated with need.

Consider three people you encounter face-to-face throughout your week. Could be someone you live with. Could be a coworker. Could be the person who rings up your groceries and bags them. List them using Table 14.1. For each person, identify one need. It could be a specific need you can see: They need a break; they need new shoes; they need a cup of cold water. It may be general, something all people could use: They need to hear their name; they need to be appreciated; they need encouragement. Then, refer to where you have enough. Not plenty or a surplus, just enough.

Table 14.1 Mindfully Meeting Needs with Enough

Person	Need	Enough to Give

How can you, even or especially at sacrificial cost to yourself, meet that need? It may take your time, energy, money, or possessions. Make note of what you could give.

Look to the needs of those around you. Look with mindfulness, not taking it on yourself and not distancing yourself. Pay attention, on purpose, to the present need before you, without judgment, to the things you can actually do with enough.

Conscious Practice – Commitment to Generosity

A powerful, intimidating practice to greatly improve the likelihood of engaging in contribution is to welcome accountability, to tell someone else that you intend to be more generous. One study found that saying it out loud to other people increased giving behaviors as well as the subsequent happiness. In fact, "a public pledge can be used as a commitment strategy motivating commitment-consistent generous behavior, which not only has an impact on generous decision making, but also on happiness" (Park et al., 2017). A public pledge? Those are high stakes. And yet so is mental health.

A commitment to generosity has three components: an identified goal, a sentence of intention, and witnesses. The goal should be simple and specific, and then put into a statement: "I intend to commit one generous

Table 14.2 Commitment to Generosity

Generosity Goal	Intention Statement	Witnesses

act each day." "I intend to give five dollars a week to someone in need." "I intend to find five ways to use my skills to help people over the next thirty days." Remember that generosity is most impactful for others and for our own mental health when delivered in person.

The effectiveness of choosing witnesses will rely on exposure and proximity. It may be easy to just tell your best friend, but there may not be much accountability or weight to that. It may feel vulnerable to share it with hundreds of followers on social media, but the lack of contact could mean a weak commitment. I suggest at least three people you have regular, real-life contact with. Maybe you have a built in group: a sports team, a church group, extended family, or supportive work environment. Those could all be great witnesses for your commitment to contribution.

Be reminded, we are not going through motions here. Research tells us that when we make a public commitment to generosity, something in the brain gets initiated making it more likely for us to think generously, to behave generously, and to generously experience the resulting happiness and well-being. Name your goal. State your intention. Tell your witnesses.

Lifestyle Practice – Generosity as a Way of Life

Generally speaking, we can give with our time, our energy, and our resources. To cultivate a real lifestyle of giving behavior, I suggest you find a way to regularly do each of these, not as a compartment of your life, but as an extension of things you already do. To encourage generosity as part of your routine, our practice is going to be partnering our time, energy, and resources with daily or weekly habits we do already, no matter what.

Think through your daily routine, and your weekly rhythms. Where do you go? What do you do? Visualize yourself going through the motions of your regular life and start to pick out opportunities to give. Perhaps you

Table 14.3 Generosity as a Way of Life

Regular Routine	Contribution to Integrate

get coffee every morning on your way to work. Perhaps you use public transportation. Perhaps you do yard work once a week.

Pair a costly, but sustainable, contribution to these routines. Once a week, get coffee for a coworker. Daily, offer your seat on the bus to someone else. Rake the leaves, pick up the trash, or even offer to plant flowers for a neighbor. Each week, add one more routine of generosity. Or, after a month, change it up.

Mindfully give attention to what it is costing you and to the human on the receiving end. They may not notice or respond. The well-being of contribution does not come from reciprocity. It is in brain patterns activated by our sacrifice benefiting others. Weave together your day-to-day life with strands of effort, work, and cost that are freely extended.

IN SUMMARY

Counterintuitively, contribution is the human capacity to expend ourselves for others, consciously and liberally, resulting in improved mental wellness. Ranging from a mindset of generosity to mindful awareness of our daily work to deliberate sacrifices for someone else, the opportunities for contribution abound. The brain is wired for generosity, with the neural connections for happiness best activated not by acquiring but by cost at our own expense for the betterment of another. The effect of contribution includes improved social relationships, personal contentment, and strengthened mental and emotional states. The paradox of contribution invites us to reimagine our hardship and our losses, for if we can reach out to improve the situation of another, we effectively enkindle our own healing and a rebirth of joy. The poet and abolitionist Frances Ellen Watkins Harper put it this way: "My hands were weak, but I reached them out to feebler ones than mine, and over the shadow of my life stole the light of a peace divine" (1854).

REFERENCES

Allen, S. (2018). *The science of generosity.* Greater Good Science Center (GGSC) at UC Berkeley John Templeton Foundation.

Blustein, D. L., Lysova, E. I., & Duffy, R. D. (2023). Understanding decent work and meaningful work. *Annual Review of Organizational Psychology and Organizational Behavior, 10*(1), 289–314.

Collett, J. L., & Morrissey, C. A. (2007). *The social psychology of generosity: The state of current interdisciplinary research.* Department of Sociology, University of Notre Dame.

Fryburg, D. A. (2022). Kindness as a stress reduction–health promotion intervention: a review of the psychobiology of caring. *American Journal of Lifestyle Medicine, 16*(1), 89–100.

Harper, F. E. W. (1854). *Poems on miscellaneous subjects.* Wiley and Putnam.

Karajagi, G. (2014). The Joy of Giving. *Journal of Human Values, 20*(1), 1–5.

Lim, D., & DeSteno, D. (2016). Suffering and compassion: The links among adverse life experiences, empathy, compassion, and prosocial behavior. *Emotion, 16*(2), 175.

Maitlis, S. (2020). Posttraumatic growth at work. *Annual Review of Organizational Psychology and Organizational Behavior, 7*, 395–419.

Merriam-Webster. (n.d.). Contribution. In *Merriam-Webster.com* dictionary. Retrieved October 28, 2023.

Nelson, S. K., Layous, K., Cole, S. W., & Lyubomirsky, S. (2016). Do unto others or treat yourself? The effects of prosocial and self-focused behavior on psychological flourishing. *Emotion, 16*(6), 850.

Niemiec, R. M. (2023). Mental health and character strengths: The dual role of boosting well-being and reducing suffering. *Mental Health and Social Inclusion, 27*(4), 294–316.

Palermo, S. (2023). Giving behavior and social decision-making in the age of conscious capitalism: a case for neuroscience. *Frontiers in Psychology, 14.*

Park, S. Q., Kahnt, T., Dogan, A., Strang, S., Fehr, E., & Tobler, P. N. (2017). A neural link between generosity and happiness. *Nature Communications, 8*, Article 15964.

Stevens, F., & Taber, K. (2021). The neuroscience of empathy and compassion in pro-social behavior. *Neuropsychologia, 159.*

Tedeschi, R. G., & Calhoun, L. G. (2004). Posttraumatic growth: conceptual foundations and empirical evidence. *Psychological Inquiry, 15*(1), 1–18.

Waddell, G., & Burton, A. (2006). *Is work good for your health and well-being?* Stationery Office.

Chapter **15**

Meaning: A Resource of Realized Significance

Adrian was nine years old when he lost his twin brother to cancer. They were born identical and grew identically, brunette and stocky. They were wild in all the right ways, "thick as thieves" as they explored the woods. As the disease slowly set in, Adrian and his brother started to lose their resemblance. With his twin shrinking with weakness and missing their trademark brown hair down to the chin, people started assuming Adrian was older. He would vehemently correct people that they were, indeed, twins.

When his brother went into the hospital and had his activity restricted, Adrian stopped wanting to do the things they used to do together. "If my brother can't, then I won't." They had been inseparable and would continue to be.

When his brother laid dying and Adrian went in to say goodbye, they spoke to each other with a sober maturity. The boys turned to men in those moments. They told each other good job. They told each other thank you. With no embarrassment, they wept as they said "I love you." And then Adrian told his brother, "I'll carry you with me for the rest of my life." To which his twin replied: "Then take me to the creek."

Adrian did. The next day he ran and splashed in, wading up to thighs. He decided then, as a nine-year-old boy, to do all the good things his brother would never get to do. He purposed to live life in honor of his twin.

Now at thirty-five years old, bearded and burly, Adrian continues to seek out and meet opportunities in honor of his brother. Even the hardships that come with adulthood he sees through his brother's eyes. He would say, "Looking in the mirror is like seeing him on the other side, like looking through the glass at a candy store. And I live all he can't have. I know my brother would jump in if he had the chance."

DOI: 10.4324/9781003521945-19

Adrian feels the pain in his life, perhaps more so because of the loss he experienced when he was nine. He feels a connection to his brother in the pain, having watched him suffer. And he has a sense of continuing to honor his short life by living in bold ways. It's the meaning he has chosen and, as Adrian says, "it carries both of us."

THE NATURE OF MEANING

Meaning is a resource that seems abstract at the outset, yet it is a phenomenon of perspective impacting reality. It is highly individualized, unique to each person. The challenge is for each of us to work with the tension between the at-times-painful details of daily life with a broader outlook of purpose. The mechanism of meaning transcends abstraction and produces positive, observable effects in holistic health, from improving mood and resilience to decreasing mortality (Schippers & Ziegler, 2019). When all else is beyond our control, meaning is a resource that provides an additional lens through which we change not only our perspective of life, but our actual functioning in it. As there is hardship that seems beyond reasoning, so a higher purpose exists beyond explanation, as if the brain-body system finds its home in a sense of meaning.

The goal of mental health is not a pristine state of being or of somehow avoiding all pain, difficulty, or upset. That's not realistic and such maladaptive avoidance causes problems (Hofmann & Hay, 2018). We may tend to avoid life, creating a circle around us that will get smaller and smaller, for indeed little ground is free from all risk. We may interpret difficulty as a result of our fault, producing shame. We may become helpless, because if I am meant to be without harm and I encounter it inescapably to varying degrees, effort seems pointless.

On the contrary, the aim is full living within reality, with the bumps and bruises that come along the way. Mental wellness is a growing confidence to respond to the realities of life with increasing effectiveness with the resources available to us all. Trouble will come. Being without hardship is not a sign of mental wellness. Adaptive response to hardship is a more noble and achievable goal in mental health. The pursuit of meaning is a response that is holistically effective.

Meaning is the resource of in-the-moment purpose and realized significance to relieve suffering and move us onward. It has implications for the brain, the nervous system, and day-to-day functioning in life. Meaning is available even in, and perhaps especially in, difficult circumstances. To be sure, there are external factors at play, our circumstances shaping our experience. Yet, the human instinct for mental wellness maintains the use of attention, thought, and will, allowing us to push back. Picture a potter raising up a pitcher on the wheel. One hand is on the outside, pushing in. The other hand adds pressure from within the moldable clay, vessel taking shape. The pressures from outside are a given, while the counter measures from within are necessary to create an article both beautiful to behold and suitable for good use. Meaning work encapsulates our efforts from within moving against the pressures of circumstance.

Meaning in mental health could be defined as an important or worthwhile quality, a purpose, or understood significance. Some in the field have defined it as "the most valuable possibility in a given situation" (Längle, 2015). It may be important to draw a distinction between meaning and contribution; too often we determine purpose by product. We are more than what we do, more than what we bring to the table. Contribution is important and I think more readily available than we realize; yet meaning is constantly present and is not directly associated with our capacity. We are not more meaningful when we have more to offer. As we will see, meaning can be found even when we have nothing to give.

Viktor Frankl and Logotherapy

The theory that meaning relieves suffering was forged in the crucible of real-life experience. In the mid-1900s, a psychiatrist named Viktor Frankl, who was working on the role of meaning in psychology, was placed in a concentration camp. For years he put his theory to the test, observing himself and his fellow prisoners withstand abuse, starvation, separation from loved ones, and loss. A clear vision of meaning altered how people experienced the camps as well as their likelihood to survive it. After surviving the war, he wrote his story and his proposition for logotherapy, a meaning-centered approach to mental wellness (Frankl, 1984).

Frankl was the author, founder, and ingenuity of logotherapy. Since its foundation, the practice has been shaped by an ongoing community of logotherapists (Längle, 2015). It's an approach that produces powerful motivation, hope, and the skill to discover some meaning in any circumstance. "In logotherapy, the client is encouraged to take responsibility for their own decisions about how to live in this world, to take action, and then to decide how they can exist differently" (Mehrizi et al., 2022). It is challenging, as it calls each of us to ownership of the self and a chosen response when perhaps it seems too difficult to do so. Yet, the relieving and healing properties that come with meaning require the practice to not be taken lightly. Our holistic systems function better and experience a more positive effect when we view things from a position of having at least some control (Thoits, 2011). Meaning attaches a more adaptive mentality with high-level purpose to keep us connected to the control, responsibility, and autonomy available to us.

Meaning Work

Though logotherapy is the official name for the therapeutic approach, daily implementation of its principles is called "meaning work," which is the mindful consideration of our meaning for the purpose of relief and healing. Sometimes meaning is found in what we bring to the world. Sometimes it's in what we experience within it. When all else fails, meaning is in our response to our life as it is. "There are no tragic or negative aspects which could not by the stand one takes be transmuted into positive accomplishments" (Southwick et al., 2016). Meaning work is the work of facilitating that transmutation.

Pursuing meaning in perhaps unalterable conditions creates a change within, both in our experience of hardship and in the brain-body system. As such, it has been studied and the benefits documented. It isn't sugar-coating – it is an integral part of our brain health and ongoing psychosocial development. Meaning is a decisive factor in mental wellness (Mehrizi et al., 2022), and it is considered a primary human motivation (Längle, 2015). The forces that drive us are established by meaning work.

Viewing meaning as an abstract deters us from reaching for it as a practical intervention. Not only can it provide psychological and physiological reprieve with similar reliability to water and breathing; it is also well suited for humanity in the context of uncertainty. Addressing meaning for a person's wellness incorporates two essential dynamics of life: the inevitability of suffering and the holistic quality of a human being.

First, we come to the agreement that some degree of suffering is inevitable. Some make a distinction between pain and suffering, with the former being the fact of harm and the latter being the mental experience changeable with perspective. Semantics aside, there is consensus that pain, hardship, difficulty, and even suffering come part and parcel with life. There is also agreement that humans have the capacity to curb that suffering, using our faculties to limit the reach of suffering in our lives (Kost et al., 2024). Often, that influence lies not in changing the circumstance but in changing our mindset toward it. It was Viktor Frankl who said, "Suffering ceases to be suffering the moment it finds meaning" (1984). Humans will face pain and may feel it more acutely to the extent to which the situation is unchangeable. Any attempts at relief and movement toward mental health must address the unchangeable nature of some of our eventual suffering. Meaning work does the job.

Second, the human being works as one holistic, living-and-active entity, made up of many interacting systems. The best attempts at improving mental wellness must address our holistic nature. Meaning work is not all in the head but sets a process in motion shifting the systems of the brain, body, and soul. Logotherapy approaches unspeakable hardship with care for each facet of our humanity. Meaning meets us in our unchangeable suffering and meets the "totality of the human being" (Längle, 2015). It acknowledges the fact of unavoidable difficulty and honors the "totality of the human being" within that very context for beneficial effect.

THE SCIENCE OF MEANING

Without realizing it, we are constantly using traces of meaning to propel us through life, to motivate us to do challenging things or things we don't want to do. Meaning is a key motivation in human functioning (Rahgozar & Giménez-Llort, 2020). Perhaps you don't want to wake up early and go to your job, but you take the pains to do so because of the "meaning" of the paycheck. Maybe you put up with the idiosyncrasies of your partner because that person "means" more to you than the discomfort in those pet peeves. Or maybe you voluntarily commit yourself to strength training, distance running, and a strict diet because of what your health goals "mean" to you. In each of these instances and thousands like them, we are able to go through various levels of "suffering" and even find it less painful because of the meaning we connect to the experience. In each of these instances, the situation was entered voluntarily, and the meaning fairly easily and happily applied. The concept and application is the same for even involuntary situations of suffering and for times when the meaning is harder to identify.

Meaning provides a direct link between the reality of our present life with significance for brain-body-soul betterment. Meaning has soothing properties and heralds either our next big move, our next simple step, or the next needed breath. Decidedly distinct from sentimentality, meaning is functional. As good as it sounds or as abstract as it may seem, the utilization of meaning is practical, absolutely boasting results.

The Impact of Meaning on the Brain-Body-Soul System

The holistic logotherapy approach, or meaning work, considers the mind through its basis in psychology. It directly impacts the body's physiology. It also finds practical application for spirituality in improving mental wellness. To consider meaning is to consider the whole person (Southwick et al., 2016). Attaching meaning to many areas of life, particularly suffering, is offered as one remedy for the spiritual need of humans to have purpose (Wong & Laird, 2024). Meaning is also noted to play a pivotal role in healthy development of personhood and holistic well-being (Kmiecik-Jusięga, 2022). Perhaps most surprising is the way the change in perspective in meaning work creates improvements in physical health as well.

One tributary of meaning research is referred to as purpose in life, or PIL, which focuses on the brain-body-soul functioning of the human. It is a combination of belief in a personal purpose, of holding individual and shared values, and of possessing an internal drive toward something. Research on PIL focuses on the impact these concepts have on both the mind and the body, without neglecting the role of spirituality. "It links the belief that your life has meaning and purpose to a robust and persistently improved physiological health outcome" (Kaplin & Anzaldi, 2015). The improvements are noted on specific as well as generalized levels throughout the systems of the human body.

Nurturing a belief that your life has purpose correlates with vigorous physiological well-being. Those positive effects are seen even when the meaning must be found within a context of difficulty. It seems that rebelling against an unchangeable circumstance increases pain and discomfort. Acceptance of what can't be changed and a willingness to pursue meaning work directly impacts the nervous system, and subsequently the whole human system. Getting connected to our significance positively supports crucial systems in the body (Kaplin & Anzaldi, 2015). From neurons in the brain to nerve endings in the tip of the toe, our entire being benefits in measurable ways with meaning work.

The longevity of the brain and overall health of nerves gain a neuroprotective quality through the existential perspective shifting required in meaning work. The ripple effects in the brain from the work are considered to have "curative" properties and "synergistic" characteristics to support traditional treatments for anxiety and depression (Balogh et al., 2021). Cognitive decline is slowed, and our cognitive reserve stands more secure when accompanied by a developed sense of meaning. Even more astounding, the brain of a person with a greater connection to meaning experiences less neurological symptoms accompanying brain injury compared to those without a sense of purpose. A more well-established PIL is associated with lower rates of stroke and heart attack. It is even seen to have positive effects on mortality rates, controlled for all variables (Kaplin & Anzaldi, 2015).

The resource of meaning also demonstrates calming and cooling reverberations for the immune system. A study was done evaluating the differing effects on immune cells between pleasure-pursuit activities (hedonic) and meaning-pursuit activities (eudaemonic). The immune cells of those who pursue meaning were notably less inflamed than those who pursued pleasure (Kaplin & Anzaldi, 2015). It is a finding that runs counter to culture and even, perhaps, to our belief. It is better, from an immune system and inflammation perspective, to pursue meaning over pleasure. Specific research done on teens showed that teens who focused on a purpose beyond satisfying themselves had lower rates of depression long-term than those focused on personal enjoyment (Telzer et al., 2014). It's as if our cells themselves are more keen to the permanence of meaning in comparison with the fragility of a rush of pleasure and comfort. Sometimes acquiring the thing we think we long for doesn't produce the longed-for solace we thought it would bring. Meaning, on the other hand, initiates relief for the brain, the soul, and the body.

Therapeutic Qualities of Meaning

A sense of meaning is not necessarily spontaneous or easily come by. It is a choice of attention, of identified values, and of evaluating with honesty the whole of your life, both the painful and the functional. Addressing these components is often part of psychotherapy because it's effective. By bolstering a person's sense of meaning, we can directly improve their capacity for dealing with stress and suffering and cultivate a mindset that is resistant to disturbances. Happiness is lovely and more available than we sometimes think, but it is temporary. Meaning runs deep and is central to identity in a way that is both resilient and enduring.

Back to Frankl, his clinical observation and personal experience in the concentration camp led him to see meaning as absolutely crucial to mental health (Riethof & Bob, 2019), especially when all the other variables needing to be controlled to protect our mental wellness are, at the end of the day, uncontrollable. Inner fulfillment equips the human system to push through difficulty. It is documented that we disconnect from our sense of meaning when we hold tightly to specific expectations of what is needed to make us feel fulfilled. A relationship, a job, a state of health, an acknowledgment, a break, a change. External factors can seem to supply an inner satisfaction, but dependence on such ungovernable, delicate dynamics can draw us away from meaning. It is perhaps for this reason that therapy focused on meaning has been seen to improve depression and mood. It increases traits of courage and reduces anxiety (Mehrizi et al., 2022).

We would do well to reconsider what we call "self-care." Connecting to a purpose beyond ourselves is better for our mental wellness than doing whatever we feel like for a day. "Self-care" and "mental health days" should be intentionally formed with the understanding of how our brains and bodies really function best. And that includes meaning and often contribution. "Neither recreation and relaxation techniques nor stress management programs themselves can fill the void of inner meaning and fulfilling experiences'' (Riethof & Bob, 2019). In other words, if your current coping strategies or mental health efforts seem to be falling flat, you may do well to consider a reconnection to meaning.

When we are not specific in identifying and orienting to meaning in life, that drive will be shaped by something else, which can result in negative effects on mental health.

> Loss of meaning in life is caused by the fact that people do things not because of the things themselves but because of some other reason and motivation which provides the feeling of a so-called apparent meaning. There is a lack of "truth" in one's activity and a presence of "foreign" motivation. (Riethof & Bob, 2019)

In order to draw from the benefits of meaning, we are required to evaluate the motivations out of which we are functioning. Are our motivations intentionally selected in line with our values and desired direction? Or are we passively submitting to "foreign" motivation along some cultural, gravitational pull? All of us will steer or be steered.

The Meaning Triangle

Meaning isn't an instinctive realization of one's own greatness. Meaning work includes deliberately prioritizing values and engaging accordingly within three categories: creativity, experience, and response (Längle, 2015). Together, they form the "Meaning Triangle" (Southwick et al., 2016). To take time to notice and cultivate each component of the Meaning Triangle provides a framework for a practical approach to meaning work.

MEANING IN CREATIVITY

Meaning in creativity is a realized significance because of what you bring to the world, and not necessarily artistically. It may be your contribution, your work, your words, or your offspring. Any way in which the world around you is altered offers meaning in creativity, even if simply by your presence and existence. Notice that. Notice where you are already creating. What you do and the way you are bring something to the table. There is meaning there, already there, waiting to be identified as such. Or, perhaps some of your meaning in creativity is waiting to be formed. So we cultivate it.

The opportunities to cultivate meaning in creativity are essentially without limit. We create with our hands: a loaf of bread or cup of tea, a plant nurtured, a picture drawn, a bed made, a dish cleaned, a quilt stitched. We create with our ideas: problem-solving, naming, planning and streamlining, business building, peacemaking. We create with our words: humor, letters, fiction and nonfiction, encouragement, advocacy, poetry. We create with our presence: being there, showing up, smiling, putting down the phone, listening, crying, celebrating. We create with our time: clocking in, pushing through, waiting well, coming home. We create with our bodies: a hug, dance, breath, sex, manual labor, organ donation. With seemingly endless options for ways to create, we find a resource difficult to exhaust from which we cultivate meaning.

MEANING IN EXPERIENCE

Meaning in experience is a realized significance in the tangible existence of our lives. The appreciation of the sun through water droplets on a flower. The way your whole body responds to jumping in a cold lake. The movement within you as music plays. Eye contact with your child with slow breaths. There is meaning in what your senses witness in the world, all unique to you. Noticing the significance of our experiences requires simply giving as much attention as possible to our senses. The extraordinary grows ordinary with repetition and absentmindedness. Long-term relationships, lifelong landscape, norms of health, and everyday rations seen from another vantage point could each be a spectacle. There is a sense of purpose renewed in the distinctiveness of each day, seen as such through experience.

Beyond lies the potential of cultivating meaning in experiences. There are the grandiose plans of a bucket list and pursuing meaning via experience: climbing Everest, skydiving, filling passports, meeting celebrities, and so on. Of the more realistic variety, we seek meaning in experiences like becoming parents or grandparents, eating a nice meal, going on vacation, and moving into one's own place. Sometimes we cultivate an experience by simply stepping outside for a walk, letting someone help, or trying something new. To be clear: the meaning in experience is formed by our approach to it, not by the novelty of the experience.

MEANING IN RESPONSE

Meaning in response is a realized significance from the human, unassailable core of our being. When nothing can be changed, our last standing option is a chosen response to what unarguably is. We are able to choose a value-consistent answer to the challenges we face. The "totality of our humanity" connects to meaning when we decide "this is how I'm going to be," and we posture accordingly. To be sure, there are ways you are already doing this, and so we can take time to notice our chosen responses to the facts of life. You can adjust or appreciate, but you must notice all the while.

Perhaps most important in all of meaning work is the work of cultivating our chosen response in daily life, even when hardship seems to be our current fate. A photojournalist captures the truth even as he grieves what he witnesses. A mother plans yet another memorial benefit for college scholarships that her daughter will never need. A business owner ensures the well-being of his parting employees as the company collapses. Dancing in the operating room, singing at the funeral, hugging goodbye. The world is full of those who choose value-consistent responses and, in so doing, cultivate inalienable meaning.

"Purpose in life appears to be biologically wired into our thinking and necessary for optimal health, a feature of our brain that defines each of us individually and simultaneously is a unique characteristic of the human condition" (Kaplin & Anzaldi, 2015). Meaning work can be stunted if we're not specific enough and can be missed entirely if we decline to try. However, if we are serious in our aim to improve mental wellness, it's work we have to take seriously. It has an impact on our whole person, regardless of circumstances. May we not neglect it.

MEANING IN PRACTICE

Holistic healing should not be reduced to removal of symptoms but encompass relief as well as a repurposing of the whole person, even amidst less-than-ideal circumstances. Trouble is a prerequisite for strength. Hardship is our common birthright. The response to struggle is not elimination but transformation. Mental health is not the absence of difficulty – it's the adaptive answer of trying, of persevering, of meaning.

Meaning is not an exercise in consolation. It is a practice of infusion. If harm has punctured holes, then meaning soaks in, filling the pores and saturating even deficits with significance. It identifies purpose in what perhaps should have never happened. We do this by using attention to strengthen the mental connection between the hard thing that is real and the significance that is just as real, but perhaps harder to visualize. **We practice meaning by aligning our mind, body, and soul with purpose in any circumstance.**

Meditation Practice – A Meaning Meditation

To encourage a sense of purpose, we at times need to shift from "foreign motivations" to an internal awareness of what matters. Using mindfulness and interoception, we will step into present awareness of our systems. From here, we will direct awareness to our values, or what is important to us. This becomes the impetus for aligning our automony in such a way so as to respond purposefully. With this mindset we intentionally cultivate meaning. Go to kristaagler.com/book/keepinmind to listen to the provided audio or follow the accompanying prompts for a guided meditation on meaning awareness.

Reflection Practice – Changing the Content in Life

Another approach to meaning work is "changing the content [we] want to bring into the world" (Längle, 2015). Content doesn't have to mean product or contribution, it could also mean presence or a way of living. Reflecting on values and how they can be expressed in daily life can be the roots which produce our "content."

To know I have meaning is to realize that my existence alters the scene in important or significant ways. When we lack a sense of purpose, or what logotherapists call the "existential vacuum," we are likely attending life as an audience member, seeing our role as passive and inconsequential. To reconnect with meaning is to realize I'm actually on the set, a character in the frame, and the way in which I act will impact the narrative. We may not get our way with the set, the scene, the other characters, or the plotline. However, you and I do get to choose the content we bring, though it doesn't happen by accident. We can select the content we bring by design and with our identified values at the forefront.

For this practice, select three values that are meaningful to you. List them in Table 15.1 and then identify specific content you can choose to make part of daily life associated with that value. It could be as subtle as facial expressions that exhibit that value. It could be ways of spending time or resources. It could be changes in behaviors. If you lived a day in which you were characterized by that value, what would you notice? Note these in the content column. To take it a step further, spend time visualizing yourself choosing this content in your daily life. Remember, visualization is not fantasy; it creates neural pathways that alter future behaviors and mindsets.

Table 15.1 Changing the Content in Life

Values	Content

Conscious Practice – The Fourfold Yes and Meaning Statements

In logotherapy, or meaning work, there is a practice known as "The Fourfold Yes" (Längle, 2015), a way of assenting to life as it is that is adaptive and beneficial. The four yeses are as follows:

1. Connection with Reality: We say yes to connecting with reality by accepting it for what it is. You may not be able to say it is good or right. You may not be able to even call it acceptable. The task is to accept that it, in fact, is.
2. Connection with Life: We say yes to life by turning toward values and relationships. What matters and for whom does it matter? Acknowledging the people in our lives and our personal values at play reinvigorates daily reality.
3. Connection with the Person: We say yes to the person, meaning acknowledgment of ourselves as we are, when we live from mindful honesty. Transformative meaning comes not from the version of me I want people to see or used to be or wish I was. We connect with the person by taking a present, nonjudgmental inventory of ourselves.
4. Connection with Meaning: We say yes to meaning by consciously responding to Reality, Life, and Person. As we accept reality, acknowledge the people in our lives as well as the values that give life importance, and engage in it all with who we are today, we find vibrant connection to meaning.

Table 15.2 *The Fourfold Yes and Meaning Statements*

Prompt:	**Examples:**	**Response 1:**	**Response 2:**	**Response 3:**
Connection with Reality – Identify facts of your current life.	My job exhausts me.			
Connection with Life – Identify who and what matters.	My family, and employees. Justice, thankfulness.			
Connection with the Person – Identify facts of your present self.	I am tired, but I am not alone.			
Connection with Meaning – Craft a statementincorporating reality, life, and person.	I can give my all as a good worker, thankful for the chance to provide for my family, and to create a just workplace for employees.			

The invitation here is to reflect on these four yeses, building up to a meaning statement that combines each facet. Simply put, a meaning statement includes Reality, Life, and Personhood with how it matters. By shaping declarative sentences with meaning content, we can reprogram our thought patterns, neural circuitry, expectations, perception, and indeed all of life. Aim for three statements aligning with the values, people, roles, or causes that are most important to you. You are not limited to three. It's a starting point. Read your meaning statements daily, thoughts recycling into future mindsets that shape behavior and lifestyle. Our specificity, or lack thereof, in identifying meaning shapes our experience and the outcome of our life.

Lifestyle Practice – Life Within the Meaning Triangle

Meaning as a daily lifestyle serves as a protective factor for our mental health. It can ward off a listless posture in the repetition of daily living. Life in its normalcy can be saturated in purpose.

The Meaning Triangle relies on the aforementioned three features most likely to frame our already present purpose: create, experience, respond. By setting these lenses before our eyes each day, we begin walking life with a vision geared toward what matters. Create. Experience. Respond. Repeat these until they hold up your day like pillars. Like breakfast, lunch, and dinner. Like morning, noon, and night. Each day: create, experience, and respond.

Create: Note the content or contribution you offer. Whether you own it or not, you impact the world around you. Choosing to mold that impact is the work of creating meaning.

Experience: Your available senses are ready to perceive unique sensations. It matters that you are the one to experience it. From common wonders to existential thrills, from the comfort of the familiar to once in a lifetime milestones, each holds meaning in how you experience it.

Respond: When all else is lost, how we choose to respond allows us to shape, at least in part, our life as it is. Frankl said, "Between stimulus and response there is a space. In that space is our power to choose our response" (1984). It's not heroics – it's agency.

Refer to Table 15.3. For one week, use the list to foster a sense of purpose through the meaning triangle. You can use the list preemptively, setting goals and intentions for ways you anticipate connecting to meaning each day. Alternatively, you can use the list after-the-fact, tracking ways you noticed meaning in each category. In the long term, the three sides of

Table 15.3 Life within the Meaning Triangle

Day	Create	Experience	Respond
Monday			
Tuesday			
Wednesday			
Thursday			
Friday			
Saturday			
Sunday			

the meaning triangle become touchpoints for reconnecting with meaning and purpose according to our values at any time: create, experience, respond.

IN SUMMARY

Cultivating a sense of purpose supports mental wellness by increasing our experience of autonomy, improving symptoms of depression and anxiety, and even strengthening our physiological health. We practice meaning through intentionally shifting perspective to the agency that connects reality, even points of tension, with what matters most. We can put the resource to good use when we look at the points of tension in our lives and regard them as opportunities to create, experience, or respond with meaning. The process benefits the whole human system: brain, body, and soul.

The meaning may not compare to the tension, the violence, or the loss. It's not meant to. The sacred nature of our intimate suffering can't be canceled out with mental exercises. Whatever is the source of your suffering, the act of identifying meaning can't hurt you more than you've already been hurt. It can't take anything more from you than you've already lost. On the contrary, forfeiting ownership of the meaning of your suffering allows that which did you harm to set the limits of your experience moving forward. Willingly, look at the unchangeable hardship for the sake of your healing. Connect to meaning in your life and meaning in your suffering. Look with kind eyes to see it, and I believe that you will.

REFERENCES

Balogh, L., Tanaka, M., Török, N., Vécsei, L., & Taguchi, S. (2021). Crosstalk between existential phenomenological psychotherapy and neurological sciences in mood and anxiety disorders. *Biomedicines, 9*(4), 340.

Frankl, V. (1984). *Man's search for meaning.* Washington Square Press.

Hofmann, S. G., & Hay, A. C. (2018). Rethinking avoidance: Toward a balanced approach to avoidance in treating anxiety disorders. *Journal of Anxiety Disorders, 55*, 14–21.

Kaplin, A., & Anzaldi, L. (2015). New movement in neuroscience: a purpose-driven life. *Cerebrum: The Dana Forum on Brain Science, 2015.*

Kmiecik-Jusięga, K. (2022). Logoprevention: A New Concept of Prevention of Risky Behaviors in Children and Adolescents Based on the Assumptions of Victor E. Frankl's Logotherapy. *Studia Paedagogica Ignatiana, 25*(4), 19-32.

Kost, B., Paterino, V., & O'Connor, T.S.J. (2024). The praxis of logotherapy: Hope and meaning in the face of unbearable suffering. *Spiritual, Philosophical, and Psychotherapeutic Engagements of Meaning and Service*, 22.

Längle, F. (2015). From Viktor Frankl's logotherapy to existential analytic psychotherapy. *European Psychotherapy*, 2015.

Mehrizi, F. Z., Bagherian, S., Bahramnejad, A., & Khoshnood, Z. (2022). The impact of logo-therapy on disease acceptance and self-awareness of patients undergoing hemodialysis; a pre-test-post-test research. *BMC Psychiatry, 22*(1).

Rahgozar, S., & Giménez-Llort, L. (2020). Foundations and applications of logotherapy to improve mental health of immigrant populations in the third millennium. *Frontiers in Psychiatry, 11*, 451.

Riethof, N., & Bob, P. (2019). Burnout syndrome and logotherapy: logotherapy as useful conceptual framework for explanation and prevention of burnout. *Frontiers in Psychiatry, 10.*

Schippers, M. C., & Ziegler, N. (2019). Life Crafting as a Way to Find Purpose and Meaning in Life. *Frontiers in psychology, 10,* 2778.

Southwick, S. M., Lowthert, B. T., Graber, A. V. (2016). Logotherapy and existential analysis: Proceedings of the Viktor Frankl institute Vienna. In *Relevance and application of logotherapy to enhance resilience to stress and trauma* (Vol. 1, pp. 131–149). Springer.

Telzer, E. H., Fuligni, A. J., Lieberman, M. D., & Galván, A. (2014). Neural sensitivity to eudaimonic and hedonic rewards differentially predict adolescent depressive symptoms over time. *Proceedings of the National Academy of Sciences, 111*(18), 6600–6605.

Thoits, P. A. (2011). Mechanisms linking social ties and support to physical and mental health. *Journal of health and social behavior, 52*(2), 145–161.

Verghese, A. (2008). Spirituality and mental health. *Indian Journal of Psychiatry, 50*(4), 233–237.

Wong, P. T., & Laird, D. (2024). The suffering hypothesis: Viktor Frankl's spiritual remedies and recent developments. *Logotherapy and Existential Analysis*, 93–110.

Chapter 16

Conclusion: May You Be Well

The phrase "keep in mind" means to recall what you need to know, perhaps what you already knew, and to hold it in ongoing consideration. It can serve as a motto, anchoring us to a sustainable approach to mental health. Keep in mind that there are available resources for your mental health. Keep in mind that your brain and body are designed to put them to use. Keep in mind that you are not out of options, and that the next step can be small and still effective. Keep in mind that your mental health need not be outsourced to that which is inaccessible or unaffordable to you. Keep in mind that there is still hope for you, your friend, your child, your partner.

The human system, with all its complexity, is uniquely positioned to improve mental wellness with what's available. It is a vehicle for the fray, not to be harbored and only brought out in fair conditions. Struggle should not be an immediate deterrent, but rather a potential opportunity to adapt, grow, and find meaning. Mental health with a dogged fullness is a more realistic aim in life as we know it than a sedate comfort that could only be secured by escapism. For real mental health that works in real life, there are real resources and practices. All that's left is to continue. Continue slowly but surely, fine-tuning the use of what we have available to us in a decided movement in a life-giving direction. And as we all, hopefully, continue in that direction, let us consider a few points of summary to keep in mind.

First, there are resources for mental wellness for absolutely everyone. Every resource won't work for every person every time. Admittedly, there are limits, some painfully immovable. Even with a focus on universal resources, there are exceptions for each one, places in the world where what should be absolute for all people is restricted.

DOI: 10.4324/9781003521945-20

In this moment, there may be those whose mental duress is monumental, understandably obscuring access to what seems within reach. I am thinking of those in fresh grief after a loss that can never be undone. I am thinking of those with severe mental illness, the straits of which distort even seemingly simple practice. I am thinking of those with chronic illness or disability of a nature directly impeding mental health progress. And I'm thinking of those in active trauma, the light of recovery not yet breaking the horizon. Though I celebrate the resources researched and shared here, I also stand in respect of the Everest before you.

Even if difficulty is not the barrier, I have seen enough of bio-individuality to know that what works for most will always have one for whom it just doesn't. Perhaps inexplicably. Some of these resources may not fit you and your unique brain-body system. That is to be expected and is no cause for alarm. The goal is not mastery of all sixty practices delineated in this book. More realistically, five-to-ten intentional and serious attempts for a given season are often more than enough. If we can find a handful of practical mental health methods that fit with our current life, interest, and need, then noticeable change and relief can come. Beneath the observable help, these resources serve as positive reinforcements being funneled to the brain-body-soul system. The reserves may vary in time and place, but they are for all people and our collective mental wellness.

Second, these resources for mental wellness are practical and effective. Still, even with renewable, inexhaustible resources, we have to return to the source. In approaching mental health with an appropriate dose of reality and acceptance of inevitable hardship, there should be no illusions of mastery. With a steady pace and humble posture, we will need to return to consideration of these resources and our stewardship of them regularly. With each new season, novel experiences, and victories and defeats we may find ourselves in new terrain. In these times, we will need to reorient and recollect the resources around us. Moving forward, we will need to keep in mind the necessity and the availability of these resources and the instinct they serve.

Third, all of these available, practical resources tell a larger narrative about humans: we are outfitted for full living and are equal to the task. Within us, around us, and beyond us lie rich resources waiting to be activated by the faculties that come standard with our humanity. We function best in a simple, sustainable lifestyle making good use of the substances of our birthright. Although we may not meet with ease and certain victory, we can find the built-in human instinct for mental wellness amid our changing seasons.

Keep in mind – being human is not a hazard but an advantage, not a liability but a point of leverage. Renewable resources surround us, ready to be tapped, and where we lack, a little's enough. The present tense moment is a constant opportunity to invest in change, relief, and purpose.

Finally, thank you for reading and considering practical, available care for your mental health. Thank you for receiving my contribution. Believing, as I do, in the power of practical mental health, I am hopeful that any attempt you make toward these resources will secure a return of investment. Thank you for your effort and for your partnership. Keep in mind, you have in your personhood an inclination for mental wellness, and it calls for resources already at hand. May you be well.

Index

For Product Safety Concerns and Information please contact our EU representative GPSR@taylorandfrancis.com
Taylor & Francis Verlag GmbH, Kaufingerstraße 24, 80331 München, Germany

www.ingramcontent.com/pod-product-compliance
Lightning Source LLC
Chambersburg PA
CBHW051959270326
41929CB00015B/2712